HCB PUBLISHING

BACK PAIN

21 SECRETS TO RESOLVING BACK PAIN

CHRIS & KARENE LAMBERT-GORWYN AND DAVID GIL CRISTOBAL

-in collaboration with-

Yves De Vos - Emma Grace - Dr. Andrea Haas
Gary Jones - Claudia R. Knights - Christine Laidlaw
Jane McDowell - Miriam Moffat - Lisa Moore
Sean Moseley - Stephen Parkus - Irma Prins
Beth Redfern - Simon Rogers - Mark Roughley
Karen Revivo - Adam Sealey - Gordon Sharp
Graham Stones

BACK PAIN – 21 SECRETS TO RESOLVING BACK PAIN -

ISBN: 978-1-8380061-9-8

Limits of Liability and Disclaimer of Warranty

The author and publisher shall not be liable for your misuse of the enclosed material. This book is strictly for informational and educational purposes only.

Warning – Disclaimer

The purpose of this book is to educate and entertain. The author and/or publisher do not guarantee that anyone following these techniques, suggestions, tips, ideas, or strategies will become successful. The author and/or publisher shall have neither liability nor responsibility to anyone with respect to any loss or damage caused, or alleged to be caused, directly or indirectly by the information contained in this book.

Medical Disclaimer

The medical or health information in this book is provided as an information resource only, and is not to be used or relied on for any diagnostic or treatment purposes. This information is not intended to be patient education, does not create any patient-physician relationship, and should not be used as a substitute for professional diagnosis and treatment.

Publisher

HCB Publishing Ltd.

London

United Kingdom

Printed in EU, UK, Canada and the United States of America

Table of Contents

DEDICATION

To our families, our friends and all the expert authors included in this book.

We love you all and thank you for joining us on the mission of making a difference in this world!

FOREWORD

Powerful Wisdom from leaders in the world of Back Pain!

Experts are to be admired for their knowledge, but they often remain unrecognised by the general public because they reserve their information and insights for paying customers and clients. There are many experts in any given field, but their impact is limited to the handful of people with whom they work.

This book we hope in part, will change that. It brings together information that would not otherwise be available to the public so that more people can benefit from this expertise. We have specifically chosen experts with a unique experience and story to share so that this information is both accessible, actionable and will support as many people as possible.

Many experts have always dreamed of writing a book to share their expertise and 'superpowers' with the world. Becoming an author however, is a significant undertaking that not everyone turns into a reality. By providing their expertise and contributing to this book, these experts have not only made their dreams a reality, they also offer a much richer experience of life for you, the reader.

We know not everyone has the same experience of Back pain and by combining these experts insights and experiences, we hope that you will find yourself in these pages and be able to gain insight, inspiration and perhaps solve your own challenges in this area.

We know that you will learn a lot from reading these chapters and connecting with these experts. Enjoy!

Chris & Karene Lambert-Gorwyn and David Gil Cristobal
Bestselling and Award-Winning Authors

INTRODUCTION

Unlike most books that you might read, this is not a theoretical treaty or fictional discussion of what may or may not work. It is real experience from real people making a real difference that can apply to you own life and circumstances, if you take action.

Bringing together expertise and advice usually reserved for high-paying clients, this book will give you insights, inspiration and most importantly actions so you can make a difference in your life today.

All of the contributing authors have many years of experience, countless successes and of course, a fair few failures. Many of them experienced challenges personally, or had clients or family members who have inspired their journeys and they're now on a mission to share and make solutions, knowledge and experience accessible for more people.

So many people want to make a difference in the world and yet find themselves held back by fear and doubt. The people who have co-authored this book have overcome this to reach more people and make a bigger difference.

If you have picked up this book and have read this far, then you either want to know more or change something in your life. This means that you, like the authors of this book, will have to overcome your fears and doubts.

We know from neuroscience and first-hand experience from training thousands of people, that lasting change requires 3 key elements: the first is KNOWLEDGE, which you will find in these pages; the second is your MINDSET, which again this book will influence; and lastly a supportive COMMUNITY.

We hope you will find this community in the stories and experiences included in these pages. By their sharing their own experiences and the stories of those they have treated, supported and made a difference for, the authors will provide you with an all-important community of support for you to move forward.

You may recognise yourself or others in these pages and we hope that will inspire you to take action and make a difference. By stepping into our best selves and living our best life, we become the change we want to see in the world. Whilst we might feel insignificant as individuals, our collective powers are boundless, so keep reading and see what differences you might be able to create for you, your life, family and those around you.

Chris & Karene Lambert-Gorwyn and David Gil Cristobal
Bestselling and Award Winning Authors

BACK PAIN

Back pain sucks!

There's no other way to describe it and it affects millions of people worldwide every single day. Despite ever-improving medical advances, the increasingly sedentary lifestyle we live in today's world along with many other factors such as stress, tiredness, poor posture and many others means the incidences and severity of back pain are increasing all the time.

If you've ever had back pain, you know how debilitating it can be. If you haven't yet had the misfortune of experiencing back pain, you're progressively in the minority and I hope you stay that way!

Back pain affects us in a way that feels deeper than normal aches and pains. Our back is the central support structure of our physical body and when it goes into spasm or pain, it affects us in a fundamental way that can leave us helpless and gasping. Back pain always seems so much worse than other pain because its impact is so pervasive in how it limits our every movement.

At its worst, back pain is completely debilitating and at best, an annoying niggle that stops you from getting comfortable. Yet, whilst physically impactful, back pain can indicate more than just physical or structural issues. As the structural centre of our body, our back represents our sense of stability and security. When we feel less secure or stable emotionally, our back tightens up as a form of compensation to give us more stability.

Unfortunately, our spines were made to move, so when our back tightens and we continue to try and function as before, this is where issues occur. I spent most of two decades specialising in resolving long term low back pain and perhaps surprisingly, the majority of my time was spent treating everything but people's backs.

For the majority of my clients, they had been suffering from back pain for over 10 years and had usually tried everything and everyone to get relief before they came to see me. The issue with long term back pain is that it can be the result of so many different physical, mental or emotional imbalances or challenges that relieving the pain isn't always straightforward.

Of course, I had a large number of clients who had purely physical causes to their back pain. The most common causes were old injuries to an ankle or knee that meant they were slightly off-balance structurally. This minor imbalance would lead to a compensatory shift or twist somewhere higher up in their body (typically in their low back) to keep them upright and in balance. Over time, the area of the low back that was compensating grew tired and would progressively tighten up causing back pain. Typically, this went on for many years before they came to my clinic. With these clients, the back pain was what they suffered from and wanted to resolve, but the actual cause of the back pain was the old injury to the ankle or knee. Only once that old injury and imbalance was resolved did their back stop having to compensate, meaning it could relax and return to its normal position. Once this occurred, their back pain would go away permanently. Obviously, this meant I spent most of my time working on peoples knees and ankles rather than their backs in order to 'solve' their back pain.

Making these kinds of changes for my clients was very rewarding, yet the most fun clients to work with were the people that had a combination of physical issues to unwind, as well as emotional and mental components to their back pain. In reality, this was most of my clients because anyone who has been in pain for more than 10 years is guaranteed to have some emotional and mental involvement along with the physical problems.

These clients came to me wanting to change their back pain, yet what they actually wanted to do was change some other aspect of their lives. This change usually focused on them stepping up in some way in their lives such as: pursuing what they really wanted to at work; launching a new business; increasing their income; or showing up for their families differently. More often than not, they were not even aware of this desire to be or act differently, they just wanted to get rid of their back pain. And yet, their emotional and mental blocks, challenges and desires would reveal themselves as we worked to unwind their physical back pain.

Whilst doing the physical hands-on work with my clients, we would talk together and explore what else might be going on for them. These coaching sessions would uncover the thoughts and patterns that were really keeping them stuck within the 'pain cycle' – both the physical pain cycle as well as the mental or emotional pain cycle they were living in their lives. It was when these thoughts and patterns were identified and resolved that the real magic happened and people started to transform their lives along with resolving their long term back pain.

That said, change is scary for us humans. Whilst this might sound strange, whatever we have experienced up until now, we know we can survive. No matter how bad or horrible an experience, if it's in our past, we know we can survive it. After all, it didn't kill us!

The brain is hard-wired to prefer situations it knows it can survive rather than situations it doesn't, which makes sense from a survival perspective. We know what we have survived is 'safe' whereas the unknown is viewed as 'unsafe' and could kill us. Therefore, the brain is innately resistant to changing the status quo, no matter how stuck, in pain or unhappy we might feel. This resistance can range from the little voice in our heads talking us down, to self-sabotaging destructive behaviour, to physical, mental or emotional pain and downright fear of having things be different.

This is why pain of any kind can become our identity – we don't consciously want it, yet the brain maintains the situation because it knows it can survive being in pain and it doesn't know it can survive being out of pain. This can be why so many people have treatment for their back pain and it feels good for a while before for no apparent reason, the pain starts to come back. Of course, there is always the potential for underlying physical imbalances and old injuries as I mentioned earlier, but having worked successfully working with thousands of clients, I'm convinced that the brains fear and resistance of change is as much a reason for long term back pain as any physical reason.

Fundamentally, it comes down to making the choice to change, and then supporting yourself through that choice with the right mental, physical and emotional support so the changes can be less scary, create less internal resistance and can become permanent.

Physical support can come in many forms such as good postural habits, beneficial exercise and an expert practitioner experienced in resolving back pain. The mental and emotional support can come in the form of knowledge, mindset and the right community. This book is a great first step to having all of these areas of support right here at your fingertips.

The numerous experts in this book, the insights and knowledge they reveal, and the examples and stories they share will inspire, educate and support you on your journey to resolving your back pain for good. Of course, there is no one-size-fits-all approach to back pain that will work for everyone. However, between all the experts gathered together in these pages, I'm pretty sure that they will be at least one of two things that make a significant difference for you. Whatever you resonate with or benefit from, use it and take action immediately so you can start to discover what it is to live without back pain.

Wishing you an unlimited and unburdened life where back pain is nothing but a distant memory.

Chris

Chris Lambert-Gorwyn

Growing Heart Centred Businesses from Passion to Profit

Website: www.chrisandkarene.com

Email: chris@heartcentredbusiness.com

Phone: +44 (0)333 987 4245

Chris worked as an Osteopath running his own clinic for most of two decades. With regular clients in San Francisco, London and Sydney, Chris specialised in resolving long term back pain. Retired from clinic, Chris and his wife Karene train Experts and Practitioners how to make a bigger difference in the world and get paid what they're truly worth. The bestselling authors of Grow Your Heart Centred Business from Passion to Profit and considered the UK's #1 Business and Wealth Mentors, Chris and Karene live in London with their daughter Mya. Chris and Karene's clients typically grow their businesses by £50,000-£100,000 within 12 months of implementing their systems.

Yves De Vos

Specialist Shockwave Practitioner

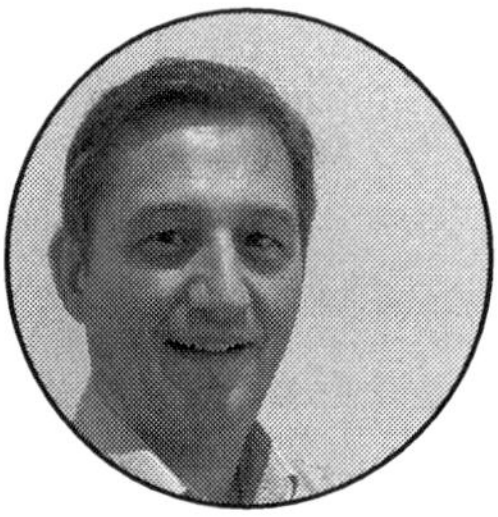

Yves has treated in excess of a 100000 clients over the last 25 years in his award-winning and market-leading business, has founded 3 companies in the healthcare sector and is one of only a few Centres in the UK and World to have the latest Swiss manufactured shockwave innovation technology.

He has developed a unique 3 step process aimed but not exclusively at women between 45 and 55 years old who suffer with hip pain for longer than 1 year and typically 80% see lifechanging results within 4 months. He works for the NHS, corporate businesses and in private practice in his purpose-built health facility and connects virtually with clients from all over the world.

He has lectured and worked both in the UK and internationally, has been involved in research and provides mentorship placements for MSc level students from several universities in the UK. He consulted in a world premiere of a health and safety short film for a leading UK Utilities Company.

He has attended lectures and conferences in over 10 European countries and strives together with his team of advanced clinicians to deliver new and innovative solutions for people with long term back, pelvis and hip pain.

Website: www.thephysiocentre.co.uk
Website:_www.solentshockwavetherapy.co.uk
www.edclinics.co.uk
Email: yvesdevos@thephysiocentre.co.uk
Phone: +44(0)2392 215 050

What If The 'Hulk's Thunderclap' Could Cure Your Back Pain?

For those not familiar with the green Goliath, he can create a thunderclap by clapping his hands together so powerful he wipes out a universe. Now what does that have to do with back pain? Let me explain.

For centuries clinicians across the world have used a stimulus to the human body to produce pain relief. In ancient times Chinese Medicine used pressure points and acupuncture. Soft tissue massage and manipulation has been well established dating back to the Egyptians. With the introduction of electrotherapy, we then produced an electrical current or soundwave stimulus. You may have heard of TENS-machines or therapeutic ultrasound machines.

When I was young, I used to observe my dad fix or build things around the house and this made me curious about how everything worked and failed. Having been ill as a child and spent many years in hospital I was also intrigued about fixing the human body. Rather than fixing my bike, I had bigger plans. What could be better than trying to fix a human body! I have now been a practitioner for 25 years and my speciality is the lumbar, pelvis and hip area. I have a team of highly skilled clinicians working with me in my centre.

Early in my career I used manual therapy and exercise to

influence back pain. The electrotherapy available was in my opinion not powerful enough to create any form of change in a human body. Then I was introduced to shockwave therapy in 2012 and finally I had discovered the ultimate machine to deliver an energy to the body capable of helping to relieve pain.

A shockwave is a high energy soundwave going faster than the speed of sound like a thunderclap or a sonic boom created by jet planes, hence my Hulk reference. Initially I used this technology to help people with chronic tendon problems but following training in Switzerland and getting involved with a group of leading UK clinicians I ventured into treating other complaints such as urological conditions and developed my own method of treating back pain.

Having treated in excess of 100000 people both in the UK and abroad and being a shockwave educator, I have numerous patient journeys I can share to illustrate my method and decided to share Richard's story as an example of what is possible.

I came across Richard (not his real name) in the spring of 2019. He was referred to me by a Pain Clinic Consultant; he had had persistent back pain for 14 years. He was a successful director of his own building firm. Although Richard had worked for many years on 'the tools' in the last 10 years he had been more involved with the management of building projects and was no longer labouring. He appeared stressed and was not managing to fit everything he needed to do into a day. His back pain was causing him problems sleeping and he was struggling to drive and sit for long periods, which is what he did for most of the day. He had also lost the ability to engage with his grandchildren and his relationship with his wife was strained as his back pain seemed to rule his life. On average he was absent from work for 8 weeks per year due to his back pain which negatively affected the productivity of his business. Richard had created a vicious circle where his back pain caused stress and anxiety which resulted in more back pain. Having been told his spine was degenerating he had also developed a fear of movement and exercise as he was concerned he would cause further damage.

Having seen multiple specialists who offered a plethora of treatments including invasive treatments, Richard had not had a successful treatment to help ease his back pain. I explained my 3 step system of how I would approach his back pain and although he was sceptical, he agreed to work with me as I was offering a different approach to what he had experienced before. He liked the fact that we would work on finding out what was stopping him from making progress and then create a solution.

After discussion we decided to have a course of shockwave therapy to reduce his back pain combined with relaxation and mindfulness exercises. We also worked on his belief system around back pain. Although the scientific evidence for using shockwave therapy on back pain is in its infancy, it has been used worldwide for tendon problems for the last 20 years, with outstanding results. Shockwave treatment is designed to target specific components of the back and deliver a stimulus to activate pain relieving mechanisms in the body. Although shockwave therapy may sound painful, it is delivered at a comfortable level and is tolerated well.

After 2 sessions of shockwave therapy he felt relief from pain for the first time in 14 years and had 12 hours without pain. This then cumulatively improved over the next 4 sessions. By the 6th session his pain had reduced by 70%, he was able to sleep better, was less stressed and had seen an overall change in his wellbeing.

I saw him again 1 year post treatment with one of his grandsons who required treatment and Richard had not missed a single day of work, was cycling regularly with a local cycling club and to be truthful looked about 10 years younger than when I had first seen him. He had just completed a 100 mile charity bike ride with no back pain! He admitted that day that he had seriously thought of having to give up his business and sell his home but that as a result of my input he has been able to take on extra projects, has more time for his family and wife and his business is booming.

Creating solutions for clients like Richard is what I do daily, and shockwave therapy has helped me to expand what I have to offer for clients suffering with long term back pain.

If you would like to know if shockwave therapy and my method can help you then take action and make a start today by getting in touch at yvesdevos@thephysiocentre.co.uk

Emma Grace

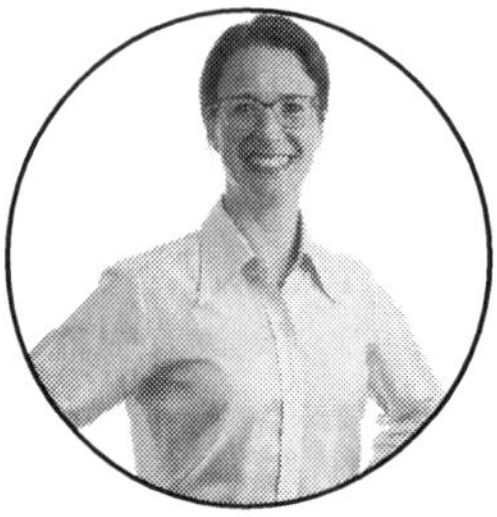

Emma Grace specialises in helping professional women in their 40s who are usually passionate and enthusiastic, but fi nd life is feeling a bit "bleugh". Their body aches, work is tedious, and their relationships jangle – and they're frustrated because they know life can be so much better. Emma helps them feel younger than they have in years, excited and inspired at work, and happy in their relationships, so their lives are transformed in ways they couldn't have imagined. They go from "bleugh" to "WOOHOO!!!".

Diagnosed with a serious illness at 22, following a mere bout of 'fl u, Emma was told by doctors that she would probably spend the rest of her life in bed. The illness took her whole life with it, but Emma was determined her future would be better. So she threw herself into learning everything she could about health and wellbeing. She slowly, slowly, learnt her way back to health. It took 10 years.

Starting from scratch in her early 30s, Emma was well but life was a bit...bleugh. She kept looking, studying and successfully working with many clients with challenges in life and health. It took a long time...but she found her WOOHOO!!! Combining decades of experience to create her own system, Emma's clients now get the sort of journey to WOOHOO that she wishes hers had been.

Emma's driving belief is that each human being is unique and infi nitely precious. The world needs the special thing that they bring, and they deserve to be the best of themselves – and well – and happy. WOOHOO!!!

Email: emmagracetherapy@gmail.com

Phone: +44(0)7392 079 646

Want To Know What's Hiding In Plain Sight?

"Things have changed completely since we met. Meeting you was the catalyst for change and to sort a lot of things out, both physically and in the rest of my life." – Clare, work placement manager.

Why are we talking about shoulders in a back pain book?

Let me ask you a question. Do you know where your shoulders are? Those flat bits at the top of your arms and below your neck? But what about your shoulder blades? Exactly. In fact, the highest shoulder muscles start at your head. The lowest ones end at your hips. Shoulders are busy, complex and often abused joints that have dozens of muscles in all sorts of unexpected places. They are regularly involved in back or neck pain, among other things, and are almost always to blame for pain in our upper back (you know that pain you get between your shoulder blades? Yep. Shoulders. So let's talk about them.

What's your favourite position?

If you're reading this, you might already know how pain can mess up every aspect of your life, from work to relationships to fun (yes, you miss that). It makes everything hard work, and drains the joy out of life.

Pain can be surprisingly easy to fix with the right approach, though, so it seems a bit unnecessary to let it ruin your life like that.

Let me tell you about a client called Angus. He had had shoulder pain for two years, and was pretty down about it. He'd spent 6 months with a chiropractor which had not really helped, so he was afraid that there was no way of getting it better, but it was keeping him awake at night, and getting worse. With Angus, the causes were hiding in plain sight. Firstly, he was sleeping in a bad position. Why does sleeping count? Well, in Angus' case, he sleeps on his side, and his pillows weren't supporting him properly. The pillows under his head were a bit flat, so he was basically spending most of his night with his shoulder and ear squidged together like he was on the phone. For eight hours. Imagine trying to hold a phone between your ear and shoulder for eight hours (if you don't need to imagine, *stop it!* Go hands-free! Your poor body!).

Think about it: you spend a third of your life asleep. What is your sleep position like? If you recreate it in the mirror, do you look like a zombie maniac? If so, you will probably also feel like one. Get some kind person to check how you align when you lie down, or dig out a hand mirror (or use the ones on your ceiling, if that's how you roll). Your head should be almost straight up from your back, and centred evenly between your shoulders. Simple, eh? Seriously, this is one of the commonest and quickest ways I find my clients get really big changes. (You will need to experiment a bit, but broadly speaking: decent mattress. Side sleepers, two pillows; back sleepers, one flat pillow; tummy sleepers – don't – I hear you, I was a tummy sleeper too, but imagine walking around all day with your head rammed at 90° glaring along your shoulder. It's not a humane way to treat yourself.)

Wave your arms in the air like you just don't care

You know how when you stay still for ages you need to stretch and wriggle to ease out the stiffness? Angus was pretty active, but at work he sat at a computer all day. Muscles generally like to move; they aren't really made for staying in the same position for hours at a time. Try clenching your fist for four hours, for example. Ouchies. But I bet you are doing something similar to your shoulders if you work at a computer, right? Every day. Poor shoulders. Move them!

Angus has experimented a lot with this; around every half hour – yes, he has a timer on his phone – or between meetings, he'll roll his shoulders and neck, or get up for a cup of tea or a wander round, or he'll just jump up and down. He has also tried standing desks, and sitting on yoga balls (get the right height – and in general, look at how you and your desk align).

Moving in different ways is one of the most important things you can do for your body. While Angus was a keen cyclist, he also needed to change it up sometimes. He needed to try different types of movement, especially stuff that used his shoulders differently. After all, by sitting at a desk all day, and cycling, he was ruthlessly shrugging his shoulders all the time, which, not being of goblin heritage, did not make his body happy. So he learnt to play. He played with different movements to find out what he enjoys doing – enjoying it is key, because otherwise you won't do it. He's settled on swimming (outstanding for the back and shoulders) and running.

So, what do you enjoy? Have a play. Jim, an office

worker and Olympic weightlifter who saw me for a shoulder issue, embraced star jumps and dancing the Macarena with his 5-year-old (both have great moves for shoulders and giggling with your kids). Personally, I always recommend yoga or Pilates – they are brilliant for the whole of you. I never thought I'd say this; I thought yoga was for dippy Californians until my PT introduced it to me by stealth, and it has transformed me – though not into a Californian!

Please note, if you have a shoulder injury or are in any doubt, check with an expert before playing.

Now, put the book down and move a bit. Stand up, stretch, do five star jumps (jumping jacks), and have a good shake. Go on! See how differently you feel just after that? How does your body feel? How does your mind feel?

<u>What if I told you that your brain is key?</u>

So far, so good. Angus was doing well, his pain pretty much gone, he was getting sleep again (Yes! Sleep!). That's a bit of a life-changer, and Angus was cheerier because of it. But there was even more. Angus, you see, has a brain attached to his body, and they both live in a life. I find brains and lives are remarkably common in my clients, yet often sadly missed in health care. We look after the body. Or the brain. But not both together. This seems a bit strange because in my experience, they are pretty closely attached, and work together, and both affect life.

Does this sound familiar? Your shoulders feel especially tense (body) because your other half has been completely unreasonable that morning (brain, life). It was also cold outside (life) so you were huddled into your coat (body). What mood are you in, with all that pain (brain)? How easy is it to concentrate on the tricky tasks at work (brain)? How do those shoulders feel after your boss called you out for not doing a great job on that tricky task (body, brain, life)?

Angus came to me after two hard years, when his other half had had a really difficult time. He had been glad to support her through it, but he was also pretty drained. He actually needed some time to himself, and a space where he was heard and supported, too. He needed time and space focussed on his welfare and his needs. Then he was able to learn more about himself and what makes him well and happy. He came to realise he also needed to come to terms with a part of his past that he was upset about. Angus is now an even healthier, happier man, with a much greater understanding of what keeps him healthy and happy. He is better able to support his partner, and has found a way to make his previously tedious job really interesting. The whole of life is so much better. And he has no shoulder pain.

So, how are you using your body, and also, how are you? Really, how are you? In my experience of working with hundreds of clients over many years, it is hardly ever just about the body. There are always other things: tensions in a relationship; frustrations at work; life just not feeling quite right, somehow. They can be big or small things, but there they are, showing up in your body. This is exactly what you'd expect, because your brain is attached to your body, and they live a life. I know you know this. We all know this, but somehow we ignore it when it comes to physical pain. It doesn't end well in life if you separate a brain from a body or a life, so don't try.

The causes of your pain are probably hiding in plain sight, things you are in some way already aware of. As a living human, with a body, brain and life, which chat and argue and change each other, you need to take care of all of them to be well; and if you take care of them all, you will also be happy. And you are infinitely worthy of care and happiness. So take care of yourself and be happy.

To explore further some of the brain-body-life issues that can get in the way of good health and happiness, Emma has written chapters in books about Confidence and Energy, by the same publishers.

If you are a person with a brain, a body and a life who wants to get out of pain permanently and transform your life, get in touch with Emma for a free Coaching Session on 07392 079 emmagracetherapy@gmail.com.

Dr Andrea Haas

Health Happiness and Inner Strength

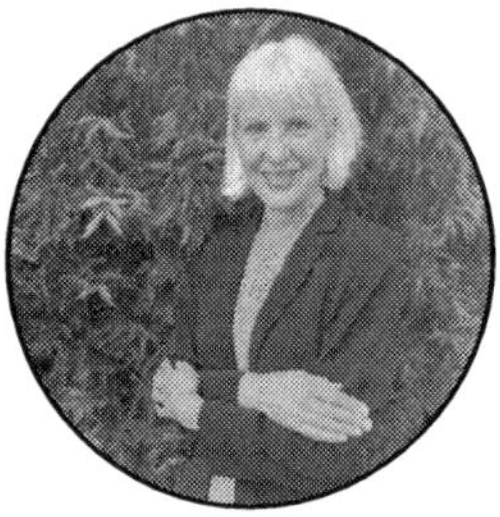

Surrey's holistic, medication-free approach to facial pain With over 30 yrs experience of working as a musculoskeletal doctor on the NHS, including working at the Royal London Hospital for Integrated Medicine, in private practice and for the army, Andrea has a wealth of experience. More recently this has led her into working in Pain Management.

Over the last 15 years she has become more interested in the mind and its impact on the body. 10 yrs ago she branched out as a therapist realising that she could offer her clients so much more this way. Using a variety of tools, often described as a toolbox, Andrea works in a holistic way, helping her clients move forward, not just with their pain, but also in other areas of their lives.

Website: www.andrea-inner-strength.co.uk

Email: andrea@andrea-inner-strength.co.uk

Phone: +44(0)7770 672122

Do You Sometimes Feel That Your Back Pain Is Controlling Your Life?

Have you ever considered that the thoughts and feelings that you have may have an influence on your pain? If our thoughts and feelings do influence our pain, would you be interested in exploring how to change them in a positive way? If so, then read on, because I may just have the answer.

I am Dr Andrea Haas and I am passionate about working with professional health conscious women, aged between 45 and 55 who suffer with persistent facial pain, making them feel tired and demotivated. So, why, I hear you ask, am I writing a chapter in a book about lower back pain? Well, often my clients also suffer with back pain. But the other thing is that all pain is generated by the same mechanism. So, the principles and techniques I use to help my clients with facial pain are the same as those I would apply to a client who came to me with back pain. Let's explore how this works.

I have always had a tendency to suffer with headaches after something stressful has occurred. They often follow a taxing day. Perhaps things have gone wrong or somebody has had a go at me. On a subconscious level it's easier for me to go home and take a few paracetamols than to deal with how I feel emotionally. Over the years, I have noticed that there was a pattern to when I got my headaches and I started to appreciate what was going on in my subconscious. By addressing my feelings and learning some specific techniques I am now able to reduce my headaches. So, what is the subconscious?

Our brain is split into two parts: the conscious brain and the subconscious brain. I like to see our subconscious brain as a huge filing cabinet where all our memories are stored, each folder containing a memory which will have an emotion attached to it. We have our happy memories, but we also have memories that don't make us feel good. Negative emotions are generally shoved down into the subconscious, so we don't have to feel them. It's like a pressure cooker, bubbling away. Occasionally the lid will pop up and emotions will escape. When they do, or the pressure cooker starts to boil over, the subconscious will provide a physical symptom as a distraction to protect us from these horrible feelings. This is exactly what was happening to one of my clients.

Susie came to see me with a 2 year history of facial pain. She had tried everything, from physio to acupuncture and had been fully investigated by her dentist. It was getting her down as she wasn't sleeping and she wasn't able to help around the house or go on long country walks. Her pain was now affecting her relationship with her husband. She was in her early 60s and had retired about 2 years earlier from a corporate job, running a large team which she had enjoyed and found fulfilling. Soon after retiring she developed chronic facial pain. She was healthy and active and she couldn't think of anything that might have started it. She was feeling frustrated and depressed, wondering whether this was what the rest of her retirement was going to be like. Her life seemed a stark contrast to when she was working. Her job had provided status and challenges, and she had been part of a community. I wondered if her facial pain may be because she was bored.

Although this might not seem significant, the subconscious can express itself in many different ways. I explained that we all need things in our lives that stretch us, give us a feeling of accomplishment, and make us feel proud. We need to be part of a wider community and feel we are contributing to it, and to have a feeling of status. We have a choice of either addressing or acknowledging these feelings as the cause of our symptoms or ignoring them, and so to continue to suffer. When I reviewed Susie a few months later, she told me her facial pain had gone. Her life, though, was also very different. She looked happier and more confident. She had started doing voluntary work and had taken up an old hobby again. She had also contacted old friends she had lost contact with due to work. The underlying negative emotions from her previous situation had gone. Now that these feelings had been addressed the facial pain no longer served a purpose.

If you're suffering with back pain or any other type of pain, you may like to ask yourself these questions:

Around the time when your pain started, had there been a major change in your life situation? A bereavement, illness, redundancy, for example?

What is currently going on in your life right now that you are not totally happy with?

Here is a simple exercise for helping to process emotions on a subconscious level.

Take a sheet of paper and just write down whatever comes into your head, as fast as you can. Don't worry about spelling, grammar, handwriting. Just let it all spill out and don't sensor it, because as soon as you are done you will shred the paper. This is an amazingly effective way of clearing the subconscious. There is something about the physical act of writing and seeing things written on paper. The problem is seen from a different perspective. Writing a journal is also therapeutic. Doing it at the end of the day allows you to analyse the day's events. Physically writing it down (rather than on the computer) is even better. The subconscious reflects, processes and discharges. The deeper you reflect, the more cathartic is the process.

If you are interested in exploring how your current situation may be influencing your back pain, facial pain, or any other type of pain, why not contact me on 07770 672122 to arrange a free 45 min consultation to see how I may be able to help. There is no obligation to this session, however, by the end of it, I promise you will be excited to have clarity on the next steps you could take to reduce your pain.

Gary Jones

Clinic Director & Consultant Physiotherapist

PHYSIO 206

LISTEN . TREAT . FIX

Making back pain simple and the solution even simpler

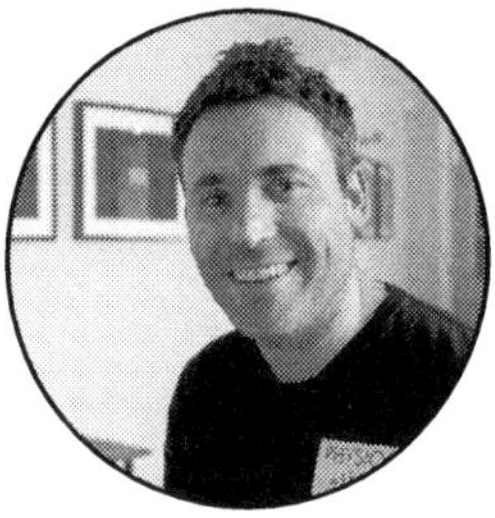

As a very experienced physiotherapist, Gary has helped thousands of people to find an effective long - term solution to their back pain. His philosophy is simple – "I will not just treat your symptoms. I will get to the root cause of your problem. This is what makes you stay better rather than just feel better".

His approach to managing back pain has "you" central to the process. He feels that this is key to achieving the successful outcome "you" want. Education, empowerment and inspiring "you" to exceed are the core values that underpin his practice.

Gary has gained clinical experience working for the NHS and private sector, many years of which were spent managing a successful private practice in London. He is now clinic director at PHYSIO 206 based in the West Midlands with plans in place to open their third clinic location in early 2021.

He has taught on courses, written articles for national newspapers, appeared in sporting publications and has featured in a well - known consumer based online magazine. He has recently been approached by 50 companies with global workforces to host a series of webinars on helping employees to work from home more effectively during the COVID 19 pandemic and to reduce the chances of them experiencing back pain.

Website: www.physio206.co.uk

Email: garyjones@physio206.co.uk

The Solution To Your Back Pain In Six Simple Words

How would you feel if I said to you back pain is normal? This is not meant as a flippant comment. I fully understand that back pain can be extremely unpleasant and I can assure you I am not being dismissive. At times you may feel like the pain is never going to go away. How would it make you feel if I gave you the solution to your back pain in six simple words?

I have some great news for you. Most episodes of back pain will get better in a 6-12 week time frame *if* you do the right things. I hear you ask, "What are those things?" Well, to find the solution you are looking for, it is more important to understand *why* they are the right things and not *what* they are.

The notion that back pain is normal is supported by the fact that it is a problem of epidemic proportions on a global scale.

Back pain is the second most common cause of disability worldwide, according to the World Health Organisation.

2.5 Million people in the UK have back pain every day of the year.

4 out of 5 people reading this book, are likely to experience at least one episode of back pain during their lifetime.

Unfortunately, we do know that 20% of people will have back pain that persists for more than 12 months. The psychological, physical and potential financial consequences of such prolonged periods of poor health will have a profound impact on the individual. Is this you? If so, the solution to your back pain can be found in six simple words:

Your body is designed to move.

Over the last 2 decades I have treated thousands of people with back pain. We know from what our patients tell us and scientific research that pain can make you fearful to move. For example, if you break a bone in your foot, we know a period of inactivity is required to allow the bone to heal. However, do many people that break a bone in their foot then decide never to walk again? No, of course they do not. So, why when people experience back pain, do they think they should avoid certain movements again? I often use this analogy, if you strained your bicep muscle (the muscle in your upper arm that bends your elbow) would you never straighten your elbow ever again? Of course not! So, why should your back be any different?

Here are a few examples, reported by clients at their initial consultation, that highlight their fear about moving with back pain:

"I cannot bend forwards to pick up something off the floor, my therapist has told me not to."

"I cannot go back to the building site and start lifting again, my back won't take it."

"I cannot go back on my rowing machine. My surgeon

has told me that rowing is the worst thing you can do when you have back pain."

An underlying theme is apparent in all these comments. Can you see it? For those of you that cannot, that is exactly where we need to start. The mindset of all these individuals is *cannot.* They are putting a block in the way that will prevent them getting the outcome they want with the negative phraseology they are using. Remember this simple quote:

For every action there is a reaction.

If the action that you take is not positive what do you expect the reaction to be? Exactly! To create positive change, you need a positive intention from the outset.

I would like to introduce you to one of my clients, David. This is a great illustration of how shifting someone's mindset is central to helping that person to understand why they are experiencing pain and what strategies they can employ to overcome this. David had been experiencing back pain for several years with persistent pain into his left buttock. An MRI scan had proved unremarkable and following years of trying physiotherapy, other therapies and injections nothing had resolved his pain. For five months preceding his first session with myself he was experiencing daily pain that was constant in nature and affecting his sleep. The final straw for him was when he returned from a holiday, frustrated at being unable to enjoy it. His mood became low and he had not realised he was depressed until he went to visit his GP. He recounts their conversation. *My GP asked,* "Do you get emotional?" I said "No".

She said, "Why are you crying?"

Shortly after this realisation David hobbled through our clinic door. I wanted to understand more about his beliefs about his pain and what he wanted to achieve from his physiotherapy treatment. The 'why'. He had not received hands on treatment before; this was something he really wanted. He had not understood why he had been given exercises to do before and therefore had not done them. Ultimately, he wanted to be listened to. So, I did just that. David recalls his first session very clearly:

"I crawled in and felt like I bounced back out. I felt revitalised. I enjoyed the experience but was extremely nervous initially. I saw immediate change from the hands-on treatment. I felt like I had been listened to and felt more compelled to do the exercises."

David had made those very first steps in shifting his mindset from a negative to a more positive outlook. This was key to him achieving the successful outcome he desired. Central to this process was also understanding that it was okay for him to move his back. He had become overprotective of it and fearful of moving it. He recounts:

"I was always told that I had sciatica and it was in my mind that if I did things, it would make it worse. When I listened to you, I felt like you were the expert. I'm doing things now I would never have done."

It is evident why David has found a solution for his back pain. Now it is your turn. Here is the solution to your back pain in six simple words:

Your body is designed to move.

I would like to leave you with this quote from David:

"Depression was the bad back. You have helped not just with my back pain but also my depression. It's one of the best things I've ever done coming to see you."

I work with people across the UK, as well as overseas, through online and face to face consultations. If anything in this chapter has sparked an interest for you and you would like to experience great results like David, please contact garyjones@physio206.co.uk to book a complimentary coaching session. We will make you confident to move your body and help you resolve your pain.

Gary Jones - PHYSIO 206 - "Making back pain simple and the solution even simpler"

Claudia R Knights

London's most compassionate sleep specialist

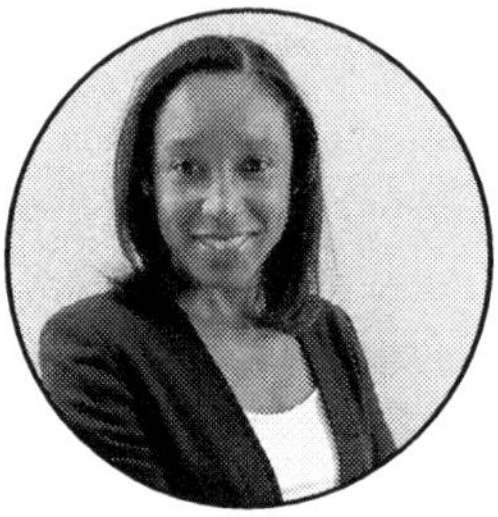

Claudia is passionate about helping women sleep well. Claudia typically works with female solicitors, who are struggling to sleep, which leaves them too exhausted to perform well at work or to enjoy time with their family and friends. She helps them regain control of their bodies and reclaim their sleep so that they have the energy to thrive in their daily lives. Claudia's unique approach combines her expertise in craniosacral therapy with over a decade of experience teaching meditation classes and workshops. She helps clients get the sleep they need to feel empowered to flourish in their careers and delight in the moments they spend with their loved ones.

Claudia's introduction to complementary therapies began 17 years ago. At the time, she was pursuing a successful corporate career when she was struck with grave health issues that conventional medicine struggled to resolve. Her journey through an array of therapies led to craniosacral therapy, which made such a monumental difference to her quality of life that she was inspired to become a registered therapist herself.

Claudia also continues to work as a Development Director for the charity, Impetus, which helps young people from disadvantaged backgrounds get the support they need to succeed in school, work and life.

Claudia holds a Master of Engineering in Aeronautics and Astronautics. She is an enthusiastic student of Iyengar yoga and lives and works in London.

Email: claudia@claudiarknights.com

The Secret Weapon That Can Heal Your Back Pain

Are you trapped in a vicious cycle of sleeplessness and back pain? What if you could train your brain to eliminate your back pain? Research shows that pain is more common in people who have persistently poor sleep. Even minor changes in our sleep pattern can increase the sensation of pain. As our pain sensitivity increases, we experience higher levels of distress. By the end of the day, we're exhausted, but our nervous system has become so active because of the pain, we can't get to sleep. We have a miserable night and then experience more pain the next day. Once in this cycle, our pain threshold decreases, making us even more susceptible to suffering. I see this cycle often in clients who are struggling with back pain or pain linked to other health conditions, and one of the critical factors preventing their recovery is a lack of sleep. So, is it possible to get ourselves out of this downward spiralling pain-sleep cycle?

An essential first step to freedom from the pain-sleep cycle is to work with an expert who can help make a massive difference by introducing bespoke adjustments that are right for you. I worked with, a client, Andrew, to help him implement the changes he needed to escape his pain-sleep cycle following four significant surgeries performed in quick succession.

Andrew's story demonstrates that any of us can free ourselves of the pain-sleep spiral, with the right support. In addition to recovering from the surgeries, Andrew was suffering excruciating pain in his lower back and down into his left leg. The operations and multiple hospital stays had severely disrupted Andrew's sleep, and he was now spending long periods of the night awake in pain unable to get the rest he needed, which further exacerbated his recovery. Usually, when we sleep, we experience several sleep cycles. We wake in each cycle and quickly return to sleep, not even realising that we've woken up. However, if we're in pain, as soon as we wake, we notice the pain, our nervous system becomes agitated, and we can't return to sleep, which was Andrew's experience. My work with Andrew helped move his nervous system from highly wired to a calmer state, and he had a good night's sleep immediately following the first session. With further sessions, Andrew experienced improved sleep for a sustained period. He gained the rest his body so desperately needed for its repair and full recovery from the operations and back pain.

I've also seen the adverse impact of the pain-sleep cycle in people with fibromyalgia, a long-term condition that causes pain all over the body. Studies have shown that when sleep is disrupted in healthy people, it produces tenderness and pain very similar to that experienced in fibromyalgia. In people with fibromyalgia, it increases their discomfort. When we have pain that persists for an extended period, our brain learns to be in pain, and we struggle with the psychological and emotional effects that result. Over time, sleep deprivation interferes with our pain processing circuitry and the body becomes rewired to perpetuate the sensation of pain. Thankfully, we can retrain the brain to experience less distress when we do have pain and unlearn the pattern of being in pain.

If you've had fibromyalgia, you will know that flare-ups can be unpredictable and that pain and its intensity can shift to different parts of the body at different times. Back pain is a common symptom. Another client, Natalie, was struggling with debilitating back pain; walking was painful, and she couldn't stand for any length of time. She had resigned herself to bearing this kind of back pain as part of her condition. My sessions with Natalie focussed initially on alleviating her pressing pain. In fact, in one of these early sessions, Natalie was grimacing as she walked into the room. Afterwards, she had a spring in her step and a huge smile, forgetting momentarily that her movement had been restricted and painful at the beginning of our session - a fantastic immediate result. However, as Natalie had a protracted history of poor sleep, I also shared techniques to help her get better sleep. I included the practical approach that I developed to decouple the pain-sleep spiral I endured before learning to manage the back-pain associated with my long-term Irritable Bowel Syndrome. So Natalie reaped double benefits from following my approach. For Natalie, better sleep and pain relief were both indispensable components in helping her manage her fibromyalgia and back pain.

A pattern I often see in my clinics is that clients trapped in a pain-sleep cycle often don't recognise the connection between their pain and poor sleep. When Lucy came to see me, she hadn't made this connection. Lucy had a dull pain and stiffness in her upper back which had been worsening recently, but she had assumed this was inevitable as her mother has arthritis.

Lucy hadn't identified that this pain was a significant factor disrupting her sleep. Lucy was in her 50s and began to experience disrupted sleep with the onset of menopause. She was always tired and struggled to concentrate. She was worried about not being able to meet the demands of running her business. It was during this time that her back pain worsened. Despite the timing, the pain-sleep relationship is not one that Lucy had identified. Our work together unravelled and addressed multiple issues that had Lucy stuck in a downward spiralling pain-sleep cycle. Our sessions released the mental and physical tension she was holding onto every day that was exacerbating her pain and her menopause symptoms. The result - Lucy's sleep improved, the pain and stiffness between her shoulders eased, and she felt in control at work. Lucy was delighted with the result and having reversed the pain-sleep downward spiral, was feeling better and better each day.

For so many of us, it is difficult to identify that we're caught in the downward spiral of the pain-sleep cycle and in today's busy world, sleep is often the first thing we sacrifice when we have a lot to do. However, when we're sleep-deprived a perfect storm of conditions arises in the brain that makes our pain so much worse and critically prevents the activation of the body's natural painkillers that help us manage and lower the pain. In essence, sleep could be an excellent therapeutic approach to managing your pain.

If you would like to know more about how improving your sleep could be the secret weapon in helping you manage your back pain, email me at claudia@claudiarknights.com to arrange a complimentary 30-minute call.

Christine Laidlaw

Pilates & Movement Specialist

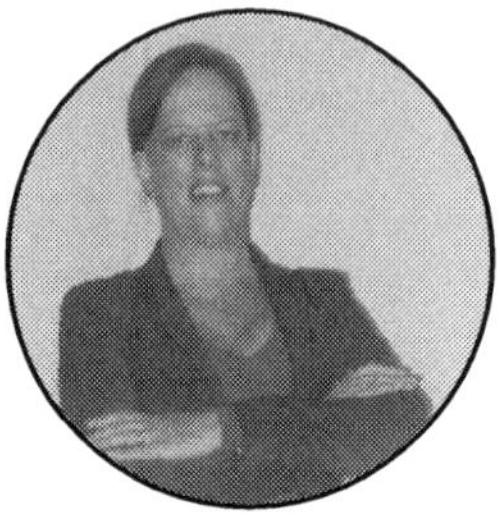

Christine Laidlaw is a mumpreneur, Pilates and Movement Specialist and Director of The Chatsworth Studio a Pilates and wellbeing studio in Cheam Village in Surrey, England.

Christine has had a successful career in financial I.T. support. During this time Christine had a car accident, which damaged her back and caused a long-term whiplash injury. Pilates helped her to recover, repair her back and become pain free. A passionate convert to the benefits of Pilates she quit her job in I.T. to train as a Pilates teacher. This enabled her to pursue her ambitions of building her own business at the same time as creating a better work/life balance and to raise a family.

The Chatsworth Studio has grown from its initial beginnings in her dining room at home into church halls and finally to a modern, well equipped pilates and wellbeing Studio. In her 20 years of practice she has helped hundreds of her clients resolve their back pain, increase their energy and improve their confidence.

Website: www.chatsworthstudio.com

Email: christine@christinelaidlaw.com

Phone: +44(0)7814 003679

Facebook: @chatsworthstudio

Twitter: @chatsworthstudi

Instagram: chatsworth.studio

Did You Know Pilates Can Help To Fix Back Pain?

Pilates is something that I have found very beneficial in my life and it fixed my back and neck pain after I had a car accident. I have since used Pilates for hundreds of my clients to reduce their back pain and get them moving again. Pilates can help reduce back pain by increasing your movement, mobility and strength throughout your whole body.

Back pain can take many forms and may be due to an injury e.g. a car accident, sporting injury or "wear and tear". Being in pain is exhausting and does wear you down over time. The long term effects of pain can also impact negatively on your psychological well-being which can lead to a variety of emotions to just feeling "a bit down", frustrated, anxious, or maybe depressed. Being in constant pain reduces your productivity in all areas of life. It may even prevent you from working.

I originally started practicing Pilates in 2000 after suffering a whiplash injury in my neck and back. The recommendation came directly from my physiotherapist. Working in the city at a desk job I found it particularly hard to sit down all day as it was painful. I couldn't lift even a laptop! I would get spasms and shooting pains down my back. I was in constant pain and couldn't dance, sit in the car for very long or at my desk! This was incredibly frustrating. I was on constant painkillers despite having physio treatment and acupuncture to relieve the pain. I started to train at a Pilates studio in London after work and after a few weeks my pain started to gradually reduce, and my body strengthen. I was going to Pilates twice a week at this point and doing lots of focused exercises that my teacher had given me for my injury. This had a big impact on my movement and strength during my working day and on one of my favourite hobbies, dancing. It took a lot of focus and determination to work on my back and strengthen it. My back and neck did hurt whilst trying to strengthen the muscles but I persevered and gradually the pain decreased. During this time, I did suffer with anxiety, depression and a lack of energy. This affected my relationships with my friends and boyfriend at the time.

After a few months of doing Pilates I started to get comments on how much I had toned up and whether I had lost weight. I hadn't lost much weight however; my posture and muscle tone had improved and I was starting to look and feel better for it. This improved my overall wellbeing and positivity as I was more confident in myself and my movements and abilities.

Over time my back had improved, as did my overall strength. Doing my Pilates every week made the pain manageable until it finally disappeared. Now I am able to do advanced Pilates classes and dance. This has enabled me to become a mum and be very active with my little boy. The success of my Pilates journey inspired me to train as a Pilates teacher and help a wide variety of clients who are injured, in pain, want to lose weight, relax, make friends, tone up and get stronger so that they can live life to the full.

During my time as a Pilates teacher I have helped

hundreds of people with their journey from pain and injury to being pain free and returning to their favourite sport or hobby. I have included two stories of my clients who have turned their lives around and completely eliminated their back pain. Here is Trevor's story...

Trevor

Trevor works in Information Technology, is in his 50's and has a history of back, neck and shoulder problems. He has Scoliosis which is a curvature of the spine and an arthritic joint in his upper Spine. He had noticed, in photographs, that one shoulder hung lower than the other and he wasn't standing up straight putting undue stress on his other muscles in his back and other shoulder. As he is a tall man his spine needs to be strong and flexible to support him whilst doing daily activities and sport. Pilates has helped him immensely to improve his posture and strength so that his muscle balance and movement patterns were much better. During a weekend visit to Prague his back locked up and went into spasm overnight due to the bed and the pillows not being suitable. His back needed to be eased with Pilates exercises to get it moving again.

After this Trevor participated in regular Pilates classes to strengthen his back and keep his back moving and pain free. A car accident a few years later made the back a lot worse, affected the arthritic joint and he got whiplash in his upper back and neck, exacerbating it. After a few physiotherapy and osteopath sessions and an x-ray to check that his spine was not damaged further, he came back to Pilates to strengthen and straighten his spine and to reduce the pain.

Over a few months of strengthening the muscles in his

spine, neck and shoulders, the pain eventually subsided and disappeared. His back clicks less, he has improved productivity at work and his shoulder does not freeze up. Trevor now uses the Pilates exercises at home and in class to manage any symptoms that may pop up if he lifts something heavy and awkwardly. Pilates has strengthened his body, improved movement and he is more confident.

Here is Anna's story and her Pilates journey with me after her back operation.

Anna's Story

Anna came to me with severe back pain after two operations on her back. The pain started off with Sciatic pain (a shooting pain from the spine or hip that goes down the leg) which started after she volunteered at a Dogs home and was walking dogs that didn't like leads very much! She also worked in the office all day at a Recruitment Company. This resulted in 2 slipped discs in the lower spine. Anna was hobbling around until she managed to get a scan and an operation to cut away part of both discs as the damage was considerable. The recovery period started and was going great until Anna contracted Sepsis in the operation area.

Anna came along to the Chatsworth Studio to see me for a 121 session to see if I could help. At this point Anna was using a walking stick and was only in her 30's! She loved to play hockey in the local team and compete in competitions. Her main aims were to get back to walking properly, be pain free, go back to work and play and compete in hockey matches! We started her slowly with exercise to build up her strength mainly in the abdominals to support her back and all the other muscles in the body too to increase the strength overall.

We did this over a number of 121 private sessions and then group sessions every week. Gradually the pain decreased and the walking stick got thrown away! It took approximately just over a year for Anna to get back to playing summer hockey which was less intense and had less training days. It took about 18 months of Pilates training, walking and playing summer hockey to get back to playing competitively.

Pilates can help at home and work if you just do a few simple exercises to keep you moving and mobile. Taking time out to just breathe and relax is helpful to relax the muscles and nervous system. This can be done whilst sitting at your desk, lying in bed or going for a walk. Learning how to do Pilates correctly with a qualified teacher is best as you will learn the correct alignment and movement patterns to help your back pain the most and you will progress further and faster without making the pain worse.

I typically work with ladies from 35 to 45 years of age with back pain, who are passionate about having an active life, gain confidence, want to reduce their pain and return to their favourite sport.

Would you like to become pain free by trying a Pilates class? The Pilates class can be at The Chatsworth Studio in Cheam Village or in your own home via Zoom or Skype. If you are in pain a private 121 is advised as you would get more specialist attention and I can work out a specific programme for you to get the best out of your sessions to progress and become pain free.

To find out if we are a match and how I can help you why not try a FREE Private 121 class?

Jane McDowell

Bristol's Favourite Drug-free Migraine & Headache Solution

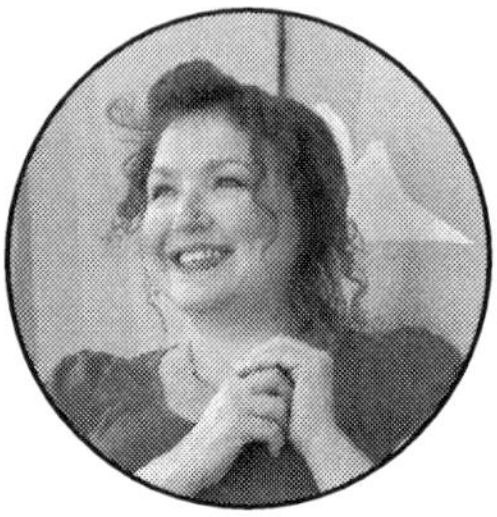

2019 winner of the Heart Centred Business Award for Outstanding Service, Jane has 20 years' experience of helping people get out of pain. Her work focuses on drug-free pain solutions primarily working with people suffering from debilitating migraines.

Jane's transformational work with migraine sufferers means that they see a significant reduction in the number of migraines they have and the intensity of the pain they experience. As a result, they regain their confidence, energy and focus so they flourish and succeed in their relationships and careers.

Website: www.drugfreemigrainesolutions.com

Email: jane@drugfreemigrainesolutions.com

Phone: +44(0)7779023117

Are Your Headaches A Pain In The Neck?

Do you get headaches or migraines? If you do the chances are you probably suffer from back pain too. Have you ever wondered whether the 2 are connected or have you just assumed that you drew the short straw and you're unlucky enough to suffer from both? In fact there's a direct link between tension headaches and some forms of migraine with back pain.

When I was 19 years old I started experiencing bouts of lower back pain as well as neck and shoulder pain. In addition to the back pain I began to have migraines. It wasn't until years later when I was training to be a hands-on therapist that I made the connection between my back pain and my migraines because I noticed the same pattern in many of my clients. Now the reasons for migraines and the reasons for back pain are numerous. Back pain certainly doesn't lead to migraines or headaches in all cases yet invariably people who suffer from migraines and tension headaches almost always experience back pain to a greater or lesser extent.

How come? In many cases it's related to stress and the posture we adopt when we are in a state of emotional or physical stress. For example, think about how people sit at their computer when they're working to a looming deadline, or someone's posture when they're driving their car and they're running late. More often than not, people will stick their head forward with their chin jutting out. Sound familiar? Well in adopting this head position we put a lot of strain on the vertebrae in our neck, we're compressing the vertebrae and this creates physical tension and can affect the nerve supply to our head, face, neck and shoulders. The other thing to notice is that when we stick out our chin we tend to raise our shoulders up towards our ears. As I often say to my clients if you want earrings go get some because your shoulders just aren't as pretty.

This posture of a jutting out chin and raised/hunched shoulders is very common in people who have stressful or busy desk jobs or for people who spend lots of time driving. It begs the question of why we do this. Essentially, it's part of our bodies' reaction to a perceived threat or danger and is part of our fight or flight response. So, let's imagine you had to run away from an aggressive dog. Chances are you wouldn't channel your inner Usain Bolt and run with your head still and your neck in perfect alignment. Instead you'd stick out your chin and you'd give it all you'd got to run for as long and fast as you could. And so it is that we still adopt this head position if our subconscious mind perceives a threat or danger whether that be while we're sat at a desk, driving a car, watching a thriller or having to walk quickly because we're in a rush to pick up the kids from school.

The fast-paced world in which many of us live means that it's easy for some of us to be in an almost permanent state of fight or flight and this has many consequences for our health and well-being. As well as affecting our posture it knocks our hormone systems out of balance, it can affect our ability to digest our food effectively, it can disrupt our sleep and our energy levels. And it can affect the amount of pain we experience because when our brains perceive a threat or danger our brains will send pain signals in order to keep us safe.

Now, it's perfectly normal to be in fight or flight mode for a short time as in the example of running away from an aggressive dog. However, when we suffer from prolonged periods of stress and sticking out our chin becomes our default posture we are creating more physical stress on our bodies and this will ultimately lead to at best mild discomfort or at worst long term pain and reduced mobility.

When my client Peter first came to see me, he was suffering from almost daily migraines. Peter owns his own business and so he wasn't able to take time off and consequently he was taking quite a cocktail of painkillers to get through the day. It was getting to the point that the painkillers were no longer working and he was fed up of feeling tired and exhausted, not just because of the migraines but because of the effects of his migraine medications. He'd been to see his GP and, as is often the case when migraine medications lose their effectiveness, the doctor suggested a prescription of antidepressants.

Peter was not keen on antidepressants as he'd heard that they can make you feel tired and sluggish and he really wanted to resolve the cause of his migraines rather than having to take more medication. As well as having a young family who he loves to spend time with playing sports; he is a keen amateur mixed martial artist and trains most days. These activities were becoming increasingly difficult because of his frequent migraines and so he came to me for help.

At our first meeting it was apparent that Peter's default head position was chin jutting out, neck compressed and shoulders raised. As well as the frequent migraines, he also revealed that he pretty much had permanent discomfort and pain in his neck, shoulders and lower back. In addition one of his hips was very tight and inflexible which meant that he wasn't as flexible as he'd like to be when practicing martial arts.

Peter and I worked together to resolve his back pain and migraines. A large part of his treatment was working to correct his posture and managing his stress levels. Happily, within the first 4 weeks he saw a significant reduction in his migraines and the amount of pain killers he was taking. He also noticed improved mobility in his hip and less upper and lower back pain. He now rarely has migraines and he is enjoying spending time playing sports with his children. He is also training for an amateur mixed martial arts competition.

Through working with me Peter now has a tool kit for managing his stress and is mindful of his posture so that he knows what to do if he has a stressful day and finds himself sticking his chin out. If you'd like to have a tool kit like the one Peter now has then please get in touch and let's have a chat to get you on the road to being free from stress related back pain.

Miriam Moffat

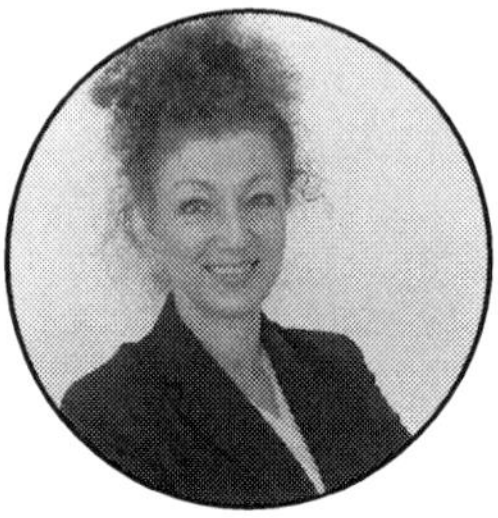

Passionately empowering people to care for their spinal health, transform their lives and fulfil their potential.

- Educator in Health, Fitness and Clinical Skills. Making learning and fitness fun.
- Graduate Sports Rehabilitator (GSR) with MSc in Sports Rehabilitation from Middlesex University. BTEC Level 5 Diploma in Soft Tissue Therapy from North London School of Sports Massage. BSc Biochemistry and Higher Diploma in Education from University College Dublin. Qualified Teacher Status.
- STOTT PILATES® Instructor, Essential, Intermediate and Advanced.
- Pregnancy and post-natal back care therapist.
- British Cycling Ride Leader with a passion for cycling and getting people out on their bikes. Completed Three Cities London, Amsterdam, Brussels, and four times London to Paris Challenges having raised almost £10,000 for children's charity Action Medical Research.
- Therapist at sporting events including London Marathon, Sevens in the City Rugby, and London

to Paris cycling.

- Registered member of British Association of Sports Rehabilitators and Trainers (BASRaT) and Sports Massage Association (SMA).
- Founder and Director Sports Therapy South Woodford, East London.
- Clinical Skills Lecturer to university undergraduates.

"I am tomorrow, or some future day, what I establish today. I am today what I established yesterday or some previous day."

— James Joyce

Email: mmoffat@sportstherapysouthwoodford.com

Phone: +44(0)7740-932496

What If A Stumble Did Not Lead To A Fall But Instead, To A Portal Of Discovery?

It happened on a 'Sliding Doors' kind of day. A sudden gust of wind slapped a wave of rain against the classroom window. The mournful Dun Laoghaire foghorn droned out at regular intervals over the snot-green, heaving Irish Sea that blended the skyline into the curve of Dublin Bay. Most of the students in regal, rotund Mr Rowan's double maths ignored the typical November downpour. Apart from Leah, who dispatched a surreptitious note on a perilous voyage under several desks and over numerous knees to me. The scribbled message was mostly illegible, apart from the F-word scrawled in large capital letters! Something to do with the unrelenting deluge making the hockey pitch knee-deep in...um... something beginning with 'S', and PE would be indoors. I dared not lift my eyes to look over at Leah, and risk incurring the Wrath of Rowan! Moreover, my dental appointment, scheduled during that very PE lesson, had been postponed. Matters might have turned out better had I missed PE entirely!

Leah and I lurched from the locker room, laughing about the note, and sought to slither unnoticed into the back of Mrs Lynott's gymnasium. Her pursed lip and furrowed brow betrayed annoyance at the forced cancellation of hockey in favour of the dreary sports hall with the peeling yellow paint and ghastly acoustics. We were late! Lynott glared at us with a look that could curdle milk from 40 paces. The class paired up as rain pelted the roof of the gym.

Now, the Supine Crab is a great, all-round strengthening exercise. Lynott demonstrated how body weight is balanced on the hands and feet while engaging the gluteal muscles to lift the hips off the floor. I raised my hips into what I passionately believed was the perfect supine crab. I lifted one foot to attempt a step forward, when Leah crawled under my extended lumbar spine to give me some additional lift! Leah continued lifting me so high off the floor my hands and feet were no longer on it! My back arched into a compressed curve which twisted as I fell to the floor. I saw Lynott's horrified face as she ran to see if I was hurt. I assured her I was fine.

After school, while boarding the train home, I felt a dull low-level ache in my lower back as I stood clear of the closing doors. Excruciating pain left me almost unable to stand. The doctor explained the MRI result showing two prolapsed discs at L4-L5 and L5-S1. Physiotherapy strengthened my abdominals and lower back muscles enabling me to participate in school sports. Cross country runs were a nightmare, but I did not want to miss out on the fun.

Often, the biggest battles are those that are fought and won within the mind. My battle was with pain. I knew I would never surpass anyone at running, netball, or hockey, but I loved cycling. The bike took me all over Dublin, the Wicklow mountains and to painless freedom. Cycling and fitness became a lifestyle that complemented my teaching job. It led to a change in career direction and a Master's in rehabilitating sports injuries. Most of my clients had long term back pain. I shared my own experience of low back pain and how Pilates, strengthening exercises and cycling had enabled me to lead a pain-free life. I prescribed exercises for each client to build strength and confidence. I empowered each one to take responsibility for managing their own back pain. I typically treated professional men aged 30 to 40 who had suffered with low back pain for three months or more. I helped them become pain-free and resume full productivity in every area of their lives. The improved core strength and stability led to greater confidence, better sleep, healthier posture and happier relationships. My clients took more exercise, played with their children and derived greater satisfaction from their chosen sport or family walking and camping holidays. I heard reports of weight loss, charity bike rides and a promotion at work, which one client put down to fewer absences and a posture that gave him a 'bigger presence' when he presented at his interview.

Now long term backpain is never only about backpain. Back pain is a crime scene where the felony has been committed elsewhere and the corpse buried in a shallow grave. There are clues, prime suspects and persons of interest. So too the perpetrators of back pain. One must search the surroundings to uncover evidence that will lead to the root of the problem. It begins with a detailed postural analysis, a thorough medical history and a little detective work.

Clients are often surprised to learn that the ankle sprained 6 years ago, or the broken leg sustained playing football at school, could be a major biomechanical contributor to their back pain now. They are frequently amazed to be given ankle-strengthening exercises when they came in with back pain. Of course, not all backache results from old injuries and more deep-rooted sources need to be ruled out. Osteoporosis, spinal stenosis, prolapsed discs, can all be diagnosed by a referral to the doctor for further investigation. More often the issue is to do with lifestyle, muscle weaknesses, imbalances and postural malalignments which can all be corrected. The STOTT PILATES® repertoire is designed to strengthen core muscles and align the spine through five basic, biomechanical principles. These basic principles enhance the mind-body connection and awareness, leading to relief from back ache.

The effects of long-term back pain are many and involve emotional and physical factors. Elite, high performing athletes and the regular fitness enthusiast, often undergo a bereavement process when injury occurs. The impact on training and performance in their chosen sport can strike at the very heart of their identity. Recovery may involve all phases of grief undergone by any person suffering a job loss, a relationship or a loved one. Once they are nurtured to manage their own recovery and they begin seeing results, real progress can be made.

A client came for treatment who had rounded shoulders and long-term significant pain in her back. She revealed that her daughter had been still born ten years previously. Subsequent tears released a barrage of grief as she detailed the horrific events of that tragic morning when her baby's heartbeat could not be detected. When my client was finally able to arise from the table, she stood up taller and straighter than she had done for several years. The burden of suppressed grief for her baby girl had been acknowledged and she did not have to hold on to it anymore.

Most back pain is mechanical in nature but is not limited to physical injuries. Our bodies give back what we put into them in terms of nutrition, exercise or posture, and they tell on us in ways we might never imagine.

My own back pain was a portal of discovery, a door into a world of wonder that is the human body, beautifully and wonderfully made. Taking charge of my spinal health created opportunities I would not otherwise have had. I cycle long distances raising funds for charities. I learned to blend exercises from the STOTT PILATES® repertoire with prescriptive corrective movements and soft-tissue treatments that have obtained terrific results for my clients. Learning how to manage your back pain puts you back in control of your life.

If you would like more information, please send an e-mail to moffatmiriam@mail.com.

Lisa Moore

No 1 Back Pain practitioner in Warwickshire

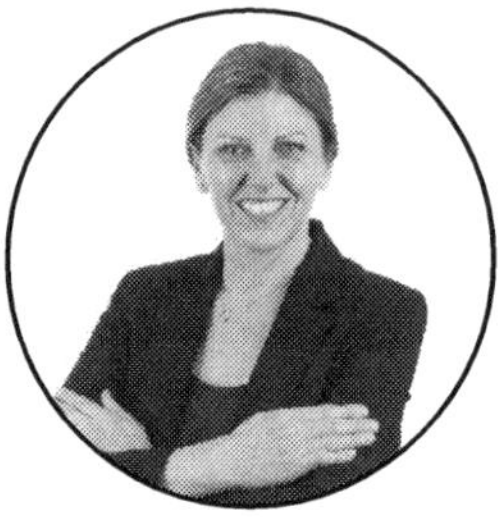

Lisa has been successfully treating back pain since 2001 with clients from all over the UK. Having delivered more than 100 lectures to companies and associations, Lisa has won the Leamington Business Award for Customer Excellence and was Runner Up in the best small business category. She held the contract for providing sports massage to the WWE wrestlers when touring the UK and provides massage at corporate and sporting events nationwide.

Lisa gets people moving again pain free. Are you interested in transforming your body so you can live your life again? If so, contact Lisa.

Website: www.leamingtontherapycentre.co.uk

Email: lisa@leamingtontherapycentre.co.uk

Phone: +44(0)1926 833003

Do You Regularly Check Your Posture?

It's a good idea to get into the habit of doing so. Just ask yourself are your ears, shoulders, hips and ankles in line?

I'm treating more and more people with back pain due to poor posture. This can be helped and prevented with knowledge, education and realignment of the body through treatment, strength training and rehabilitation.

Many years ago I was working in the corporate world, sitting at an office desk over a PC. The pain that I endured with my back was unbelievable. Tight upper back muscles hard as a board, constant headaches and lower back pain from slouching. I would admire the few I met with an upright and relaxed posture, and ask myself, 'How do you get a posture like that?' I'd developed an interest in health, wellness and the human body (which led me to my career change a few years later) and was reading an article about habits, behaviour and muscle memory. Did you know it takes an average of 66 days for a new behaviour to become automatic? Great, I thought to myself, I'm going to start with my first wish, to be able to sit down without crossing my legs. I put a post-it note on my computer screen which read 'uncross legs'. Whenever I crossed my legs I'd see this and uncross them. It wasn't too long before this habit became automatic.

Soon after I was implementing others in the same manner to help me improve my posture. Unhappiness in my career was slowly eating away at me physically, mentally and emotionally and I was taking my unhappiness out on those around me. Finally I decided to take the plunge and do a course that would lead me to my desired career. Now I have my own thriving business in Leamington Spa with associates working from my clinic, We help others with back pain and teach them how they can correct their problems themselves.

This generation has a seen a big shift in work practice with an increased use of technology or spending hours in a car travelling long distances. Even furniture is made for slouching. All of these lifestyle changes have altered our posture. From an upright back with shoulders down to a slouched lower back, with rounded shoulders that creep up to our ears, a hunched upper back with head and neck extended forward; known as 'Tech Neck'.

Poor posture can lead to

- Back pain
- Headaches
- Migraines
- Intermittent nerve pain (numbness, tingling) in the arm and fingers
- Pain between the shoulders blades and spine
- Pain from the top of the shoulder blade into the base of the head

- Pain along the length of the spine especially when touching chin to chest

Getting into the habit of checking your posture throughout the day can help with developing your new one.

- Sit on your sitting bones. This will tilt the top of your pelvis slightly forward bringing the shoulders and head back and engage the core muscles.
- Make sure your ears are in line with your shoulders. This will take pressure off the neck. For every inch where your head moves forward from the shoulders, the weight of the head increases by at least 10 pounds. (The head is as heavy as a bowling ball.)
- Keep your shoulders down and back. This will prevent tension in the upper back, which can creep up into the neck and cause headaches.
- Sit tall. This helps create space between the vertebra of the spine allowing movement without restriction and helps to strengthen the muscles of the spine and core.
- When sat at your workstation support your arms on the desk and keep elbows, hips, knees and ankles between 110 and 90 degrees.

When standing

- Keep your feet flat on the floor so your weight is equally distributed through your body.
- Make sure your ears, shoulders, hips and ankles are in line. This will keep you balanced and your

posture will feel effortless.

- Keep your shoulders down and back. If they are then they're not causing tension to build up in the upper back and neck.
- Stand tall. This helps create space between the vertebra of the spine allowing movement without restriction and helps to strengthen the muscles of the spine and core.

'Remember, muscle has memory. The more times you correct your posture the more chance of it staying corrected', is something I always say to my clients. Client A came to see me with chronic pain in her upper back which she'd endured for months, thinking it would go away. She had migraines on a daily basis, discomfort in her neck which prevented her from sleeping and intermittent pain down her arms and into her fingers which occasionally were numb. Her GP had referred her to a consultant for repetitive strain injury. She was in a high-powered job sat at a desk all day and she was finding it difficult to concentrate. Her productivity had reduced and she was afraid of not reaching her targets. More to the point, she was afraid of not providing for her family. Her poor posture was causing physical stress and all she could focus on was the pain which then caused her mental stress. Her high workload was causing mental stress and because she was sitting for long periods of time this was then causing her physical stress. Her back was so painful to touch that the first session was just to introduce her muscles to the changes they were about to go through. With an exercise plan in place and advice on how to set up her workstation she noticed a big difference after just one treatment. With still a long way to go we went on a journey together to eliminate the pain, even the numbness in her fingers (as it wasn't a repetitive strain injury). Exercises were given to realign and strengthen her posture and I educated her on the things she could do to help herself. Within a short period of time we had eliminated all of her symptoms and she was back enjoying her work and family life again pain free.

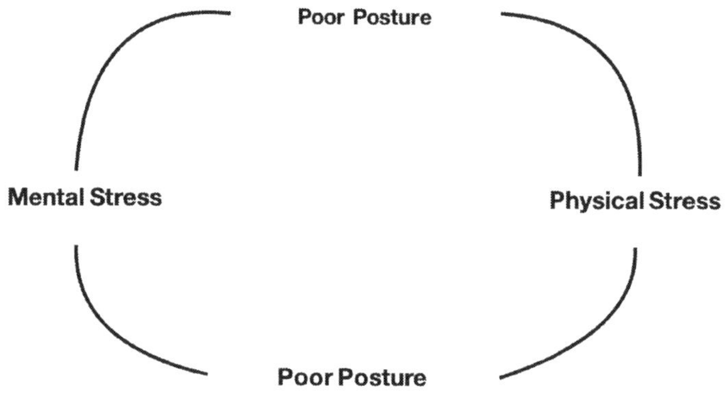

5 Top tips to beat back pain.

- Remember to ask yourself throughout the day 'How am I sitting/standing?' Run through the checklist of ears, shoulders, hips and ankles.
- Sit on your sitting bones and engage your core muscles,
- Put a post-it note on your PC/laptop/dashboard to remind you of your posture,
- Rebalance with yoga or Pilates; it will stretch and strengthen your muscles,
- Have a regular maintenance massage.

After years of back pain and seeing lots of different

specialists from chiropractors and acupuncturists to physiotherapists, who haven't been able to relieve me of my aches and pains, Lisa has been working her magic on me for the last 4 weeks and my pain has greatly reduced from the first session. I feel very confident in Lisa's skills and I'm very grateful we crossed paths. If you suffer with back pain, I highly recommend a visit to Lisa.

Liz Wood

After two appointments with Lisa my condition greatly improved and my movement is now 100% better, I would strongly recommend anyone with back pain see Lisa as she is extremely thorough and effective with her results.

John Wills

Sean Moseley

The South Coast solution to knee pain

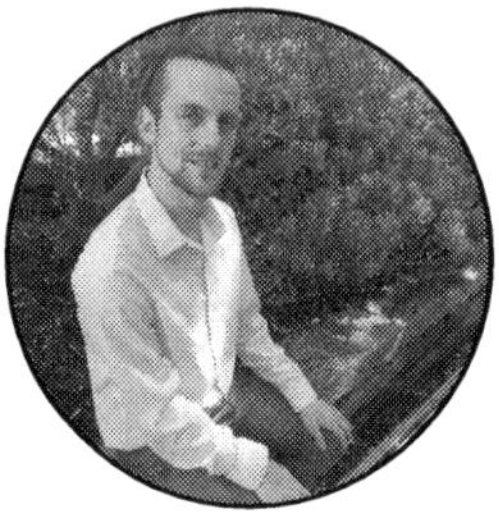

Having personally battled his way through injury to success on the basketball court, Sean has spent over 12 years in the world of health and fitness. After starting his successful business immediately upon graduation from University Sean has worked with clients ranging from professional athletes to sedentary office workers.

Sean found his passion in working with men whose pain is preventing them from being the fun superhero Dad that they envisioned of themselves, he takes the frustrations from pain and turns it into a drive to create pain free memories.

Email: Hello@seanmoseley.com

Phone: +44(0)7983107033

Is Pain Holding You Back? What If I Told You The Mind And Movement Is The Key?

If the answer to the above question is yes, then high five because we've both been in the same boat, and big hugs because perhaps you're still in this rocky boat. I'm Sean Moseley, The South Coast solution to knee pain and I help dads to be free from pain when playing with their children. Yes, I know, a mention of a knee in a book for back pain, what's going on? There's a link, trust me.

Let me start by telling you about my journey with back pain, and then I'll link that to my top tips to beat back pain. It starts with me developing a passion for basketball at the age of 12. My tutor at school suggested I should go to a taster session for some extracurricular activity (Thankyou Mr Bowles). I signed up for school trials and I felt it went well, but disaster! I didn't make the cut, and this really (Insert expletive of your choice) riled me up. This lit a burning passion inside me to succeed at basketball. Throughout the summer my Dad took me to a court to help me train; for this he's an absolute champion due to suffering with back pain at the time himself. Towards the end of the summer I'd joined a local league team and had been successful in national league trials. Upon the first day back at school I felt smug as I told Mr Bowles I was now a national premier league basketball player.

Now picture the scene, It's one of my first away games for national premier league, I'm playing away in London, excited, warmed up, ready to check into the game. "Sean lets go", they said.

This is it! I thought, *My time to shine*. The ball is passed my way, a defender tips the ball loose, it's rolling along the floor heading out of bounds and I dive for it! Then I feel searing pain, my world of excitement is suddenly a world of pain, fear and lack of breath. What's going on? Why can't I breathe? Is this the end? Fear, such fear! Unbeknown to me an opposing player had also dived for the ball, all 6ft 4 of him came crashing down onto my small 5ft 6 frame, landing directly on my back, squeezing the air from me.

This was the beginning of debilitating back pain between the ages of 14-17, resulting in many missed games, missed training sessions and missed P.E. lessons. I was feeling totally let down by my body and unable to participate in the one thing I felt passionately about; basketball! It felt like every time I began to make progress the back pain would return. How many of you can associate with this? The pain starts to loosen its grips and returns as bad as before?

I'd seen many therapists during that time; I'd been cracked, poked, needled and massaged more times than I care to think about. I would do my exercises, feel strong again, get back to training for a couple of months and be thrown right back to square one. Utilising my knowledge as an expert, I now understand the recurring issues ultimately came down to not being able to recognise what had happened at the root cause of the pain; the emotional trauma that came with feeling so scared in my place of fun (The basketball court). Without recognising I needed to teach myself basketball is safe, true recovery (body and mind) could not occur, and without recovery, I certainly would not have been able to revitalise my life, no matter how hard I trained or how many times I was poked and prodded. Does this make sense? Allow me to explain it in a different way. Pain is an experience in the same way that having fun is an experience. There are many things that factor into the experience of having fun; the activity we're doing, how tired we are, the people we're around etc. Pain is the same way; it's influenced by many factors; sleep, diet, alcohol, smoking, exercise, emotions, emotional blocks, stress etc.

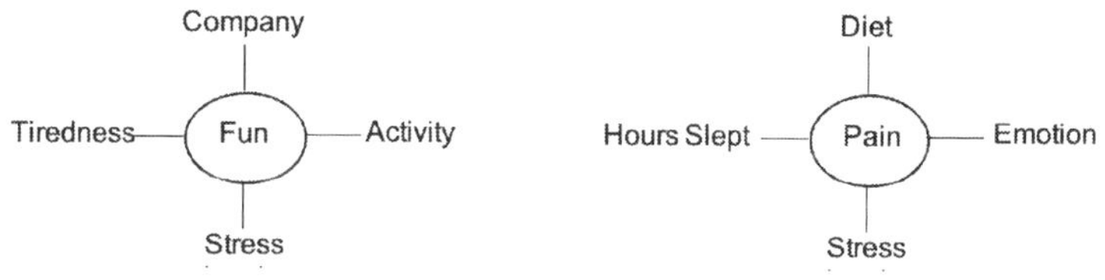

Action Step: Create your own pain spider diagram using the power of recognition.

The key role of the brain is to keep us alive, and it's done an amazing job; I'm here to write this chapter, and if you're reading this, it also means yours has done a great job too. However, my brain had learned a behaviour that if I took a knock on the basketball court this could mean I lose the ability to breathe, therefore basketball is 'dangerous' and must be avoided. Once my brain had linked those two things together, it learned an avoidance strategy of 'back pain = I stop playing'. Well done brain, you kept me safe, thank you! (How many of us thank our brains for keeping us safe? I bet not many right? And that's okay, but showing ourselves love is absolutely vital!) However, this avoidance strategy wasn't conducive to me participating in what I'm passionate in. When we can recognise certain behaviours like this, we can teach the brain new behaviours, a big part of this with pain is teaching the brain that it's okay and safe to move; remember 'rest is rust, and motion is lotion'! "But Sean", I hear you say, "When I move it hurts, so I must be doing more damage". Think about the experience of pain we just discussed; pain isn't all about what's happening directly at the site of pain. I will also add that numerous recent scientific studies have indicated that levels of pain HAVE ABSOLUTELY NO CORRELATION to the damage of our bodily structures. Therefore, when we're in pain, it's vital that we find a way to move. Even if it's the smallest movements at first this is totally okay. Do the scary thing day after day, to create permanent changes going forward.

Do you remember at the start of this chapter, I mentioned there can be a link between backs and knee pain? I also learned this the hard way due to my avoidance mechanisms. My back had become very stiff, and at the same time I'd started to regularly get knee injuries and knee pain. This reached a crescendo when I tore a ligament in my right knee during pre-season for my final u18 premier league season. Unbeknown to me at the time, if we're lacking movement in our backs, our hips and knees have to take the brunt of this. The increased rotation at the hips puts our knees under so much more pressure.

To summarise, my top tips for back pain are;

- Recognise what worsens your pain and take charge of these areas of your life.
- Rest is rust, and motion is lotion.
- Remember, exercise is like medicine; like medicine we prefer it to taste good, therefore find a way to move which you find fun.
- Gradually reintroduce movements that are scary for you now.
- Listen to what your body is telling you and resolve the issue, when we ignore it other parts of the body take the brunt.
- Avoid changing your posture to accommodate pain as this can become a more long-term adaptation, a postural shirt such as what I've used from ActivePosture®.

I'm thankful for these tribulations. It was during this time of repairing my knee that I gained a love of the knee itself. I don't think I would have the pleasure of being able to change people's lives today if I hadn't gone through these bumps in my journey. As I mentioned earlier in my story, my Dad always pushed himself through his pain to play basketball with me at the park. This is superhero behaviour in my opinion. The fact that parents will push themselves through pain for the betterment of their children is such a beautiful act of love, therefore I've made it my mission to give as many dads throughout my lifetime the opportunity to create pain free memories playing with their child. If you're curious and would like to learn more, email me at hello@seanmoseley.com for a free back pain mobility download.

Stephen Parkus

Making back pain just a memory

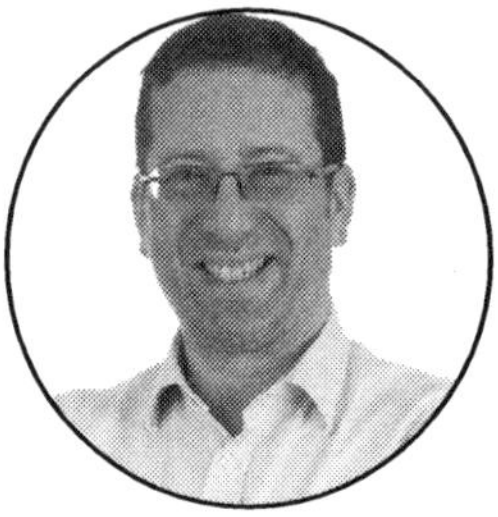

Stephen has helped thousands of clients become free from back pain over 20 years in healthcare, and regularly lectures to GPs, Education Professionals and Personal Trainers on back pain and hypermobility.

He is often called upon to give second opinions to clients. Stephen changes his clients' belief in what their bodies are capable of, helping them out of pain, towards more energy and a more fulfilled life.

Website: www.stephenparkus.com

Email: stephen@stephenparkus.com

Phone: +44(0)2087 280 625

Have You Accepted Back Pain As Part Of Your Life?

Have you been told that you shouldn't have back pain, that it's all in your head?

Have you been told that you are stuck with your back pain, that nothing will help?

What if you could do something about it?

At school, I was always interested in exercise, played rugby and got into weightlifting. In my late teens, I had two episodes of severe back pain, which came as a shock as I had never had pain before. The pain came without warning, during a summer job. Thankfully the pain didn't last more than a few days each time, but I couldn't find any useful advice to guide me, so I never knew what caused it, or whether I should worry that it might come back.

Whilst studying engineering at University, I developed an interest in Yoga, Tai Chi and Shiatsu massage, and found I had a talent in using my hands to relieve pain and ease stress through the use of these techniques. I loved doing this, and eventually decided it was time for a career change. After studying for a massage diploma, then qualifying as a Physiotherapist, I finally felt I could help people. Working in the NHS, I often felt that I did not have enough time with patients to use all my skills. My engineering background gave me a good eye for spotting problems with alignment to help people's posture. I could then use my hands, and also give advice on exercise and lifestyle to reduce further strain on their backs. After gaining a few other skills along the way, I left the NHS to start my private practice in 2008 and developed my own approach; since then it has been my honour to help thousands of clients.

Since starting my own practice, I have had many experiences with different patients, including my own daughter. She is in her late teens, and like me, has experienced neck and back pain, as have some of her friends. They have spoken of similar challenges in trying to find help but not finding an answer. Recognising the increasing tendency in this age group towards poor posture often caused by screen usage, I have developed a keen interest in treating clients of a similar age to my daughter, and of the age I was when I had back pain, to help them reclaim some energy and enjoyment in their lives.

I typically work with women in their late teens and early 20s with at least 1 year of back pain, which is affecting their ability to work, sleep and enjoy life. I help them to relieve their pain, sleep better and have more energy, perform better at work and live life to the fullest.

Treating back pain is both an art and a science, to put the body into balance. The cause of the pain can be from a lack of muscle balance, meaning some muscles are too tight or not strong enough, and this can often affect posture.

Sometimes people try to help themselves but do the right thing at the wrong time or in the wrong way, and find that what they expect to help does not work.

Additionally, people often worry that what they need to do to fix their problem will take too much time or energy, or believe they are beyond help.

An example is one of my patients, a 25-year-old woman, working in retail and also helping care for her disabled mother. She had almost given up hope of finding an answer. She had 10 years of low back pain, had gained weight, and thought she would have pain for life. She was depressed by her back pain, feared exercise in case it made her pain worse, had low energy and slept badly, and had low self-esteem and confidence. I helped to relieve her pain using some hands-on methods, and advised on how to improve her posture. I also gave her some very gentle exercises to start the process of change, and showed her how to help her mother without straining herself. She recovered from her back pain, started to sleep better and have more energy, and had more self-esteem and confidence. As a result of this, many new choices were available to her, since she was no longer struggling with this pain.

For those who are young and otherwise healthy, the cause of their back pain often isn't obvious at first glance, and therefore it can seem as if there is no reason for their pain.

A good example is another of my patients, a healthy and fit 17-year-old student and keen long-distance swimmer, who developed low back pain as she increased her training for a charity event swimming across the Channel. Her low back pain prevented her from training properly and she feared she would miss the event and let down her team-mates. Although she was fit, strong and flexible, my unique assessment approach revealed that she was also out of balance. After working with her to restore her balance, with just a few extra exercises, she reported that her back pain had disappeared, she could swim faster and was less tired, and participated in the event with her team.

A common cause of back pain is poor posture from long hours in front of a computer. Even if you think you are sitting straight at your computer, check every hour, and if you have slumped, then sit up straight again. This will gradually get easier!

People who work at a computer can also often develop tight hips, which can then cause low back pain when standing. If you have this, try these simple daily exercises:

- Lie on your back on your bed, with both legs straight out.
- Pull one knee towards your chest, hold the knee with your hands and hold for 10 seconds.
- Then release your knee and straighten out your leg resting it back on the bed.
- Repeat this movement with your other leg.
- Repeat on each leg 3 times.
- Then pull both knees towards your chest at the same time and hold for 10 seconds, then release. Repeat this 3 times.

Are you fed up with not getting an answer for your back pain, or for someone in your family?

Would you like enough time to fully work out the problem, and not feel rushed with advice that doesn't quite work for you?

Please email me at Stephen@stephenparkus.com to

request a copy of my free back pain exercise e-book, to start the road to your recovery.

If you would like to find out more, please email me at Stephen@stephenparkus.com to book a free discovery session online, or at my clinic in North West London.

Wishing you good health and a healthy back.

Irma Prins

Helping kids move freely

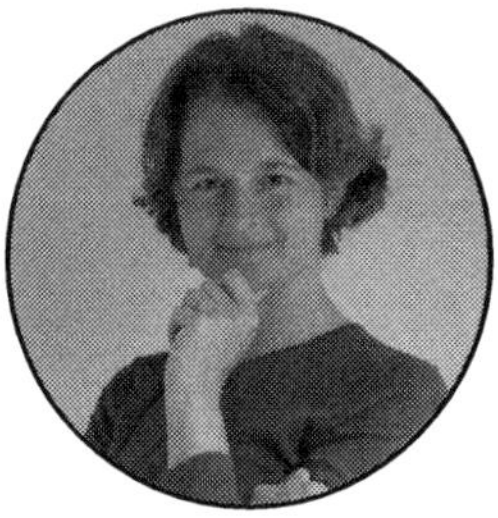

Irma has been unlocking people's energy by helping them to move the way they are designed to for 3 decades now. When she started applying her physiotherapy skills to young children, whilst they were positioned on a walking horse (hippotherapy/ equine facilitated physiotherapy), she was amazed about how much progress they made in their development and how quickly they achieved it. Since then she has been keen to see as many children benefit from this as possible.

Therefore, she has helped shape the future of hippotherapy/ equine facilitated therapy and the education of therapists through her roles in the committee of the Chartered Physiotherapists in Therapeutic Riding and Hippotherapy (CPTRH), UK. She has served on this Specialist Interest Group for 8 years. She also took part in the first European Equine Facilitated Therapy Network meeting in Prague in 2019, where decisions were made about the definition of Equine Facilitated Therapy, and a plan was developed on how to bring all the expertise in Europe together under one umbrella. Irma runs lectures for other professionals.

Irma is based in the Midlands, UK and expanding! Out of area? Don't worry. Sessions without horses can be done on-line.

Email: irma@irmaprins.com

Facebook: FreedomPhysioServices

Phone: +44(0)7402 825 904

Why Let Your Horse Suffer From Your Injury?

Do you have back pain when you are horse riding? Is this stopping you from enjoying your horse?

The flexibility and function of the horse's joints are very important for the comfort and movement of the horse as well as that of the rider. If the horse is not supple, or is in pain, the experienced rider usually knows it. Because riders don't like to see their animals suffer, they let their horses be checked regularly by a professional. Did you know the reverse is also true? That the rider's abilities and injuries also have an effect on the horse's comfort and movement? If a rider is in pain and braces her back to protect herself, she also blocks the movement in the horse's spine. However, does the rider let him or herself be checked? When was the last time you had a 'service'? Many riders have had injuries in the past, which leave some issues in their bodies they don't even know about.

Let me give you an example. Sam had been riding since she was little. She had fractured her ankle a long time ago which had left her with some stiffness in her foot. Although still young, she also suffered from arthritis in her lower back, due to a fall when she was a teenager. For her job she had to train horses, and riding them made her uncomfortable. When I assessed Sam, I found that her lower back was stiff and she was unable to move her pelvis freely. This made her sit a bit slumped on her horse. Let me expand a little on this to help you understand. The bottom of the spine consists of 5 bones stacked on top of each other which should be able to bend forwards, backwards and sideways from each other and rotate to the left and right. Are you able to move to the left and the right an equal amount? When a person has had a back injury this movement often doesn't return by itself and the supporting muscles are usually weak.

I gave Sam exercises to do so she could start building these muscles up again and I taught her how to increase the suppleness of her back joints and, most importantly, how to coordinate the movements between them. Suppleness and coordination are important factors when riding, because these allow you to stay in tune and balance with the horse's movements. We also addressed the stiffness in Sam's foot.

To do this we used a 3 step system. In general, when doing work on the ground to identify and resolve an issue in the body:

- Step 1 It is important that the person is then also able to integrate this into her riding and learns to fine tune the new movement
- Step 2 After this phase it is a case of strengthening the new abilities by adding increasingly greater challenges
- Step 3 New habits become established and the client can use them in unexpected situations, which ultimately makes her a safer rider

When using this 3 step system with clients, the results

are better the more time is spent establishing the new skills.

Let's look at the rest of Sam's journey through the steps. When Sam was through the first phase of solving the issue of her stiffness, we went to the second phase of learning to use this newfound movement in the activities she needed. She learned to control the movements on the gym ball and on her own saddle placed on a saddle horse. I like using these steps because the rider can then concentrate on her own body first, without having to worry about where the horse is going.

We ensured that the seat bones were placed in the right place on the saddle so her pelvis could move freely. We also ensured that the feet were positioned with the ball of the foot on the stirrup iron. That is why we need supple ankles. A correct foot position allows the pelvis to land in the right place of the saddle and not towards the back, so the horse's back doesn't receive unnecessary pressure.

The saddle horse allowed Sam to practice equal weight going down through her left and right seat bones. Usually the rider is more aware of one of these and the horse often veers to this side. A way to check if you sit equally on both sides is to move your hands under your buttocks and feel the pressure of the bones into your hands. Is it equal? If not, are you able to correct this? When there was equal weight through both seat bones, Sam could use the 'bucket' exercise. She would imagine her pelvis was a bucket full of water. This meant that she would tilt her pelvis forward to spill the water over the front rim of the bucket and backwards for the reverse. The challenge was to keep her upper body still throughout.

Next we transferred this skill to the horse. When on the horse it is helpful to let the horse move the pelvis of the rider initially. It helps the person's back to warm up and to get a feel for the horse's movements. So with her seat bones in place Sam let them follow the horse, while letting the water spill in front and behind. Once she had mastered this, she concentrated on moving the water over the sides of the bucket and letting her legs relax. Once she was familiar with moving fluidly with the horse, she practised controlling the range by making the movement smaller and bigger. This way she could learn to control the speed and rhythm of the horse. Does this sound like something you would like to be able to do?

Sam was now ready for the third stage: to strengthen this control by giving her more challenging situations to practise. These were moving at higher speeds of the horse and using the legs to give instructions to the horse etc. On our fifth session together, Sam told me that her colleagues had noticed that she had a better posture while riding. Sam also didn't experience back pain anymore, during or afterwards. When she rode she looked more balanced and safer. The horse moved with more suppleness and was able to bring his hind legs further forward. This is important for the carrying abilities of the horse and a foundation for all disciplines in the riding world.

So resolving the movement issues of the rider and then helping her to integrate this into all her riding challenges makes the rider more effective, comfortable and safe, and it allows the horse to move with more ease and grace. I really enjoy watching this transformation happening between horse and rider. Are you ready to work on your body so your horse and you can both feel free to move?

If so, please contact me on irma@irmaprins.com or phone 07402 825904 to arrange a free 1 hour consultation, in which we find out what your areas for improvement are and what the best way forward is to address them. Consultations are offered in person or remotely on-line. Book your appointment now and start enjoying pain free horse riding!

Beth Redfern

Helping people with long term back pain get out of pain and confident about moving

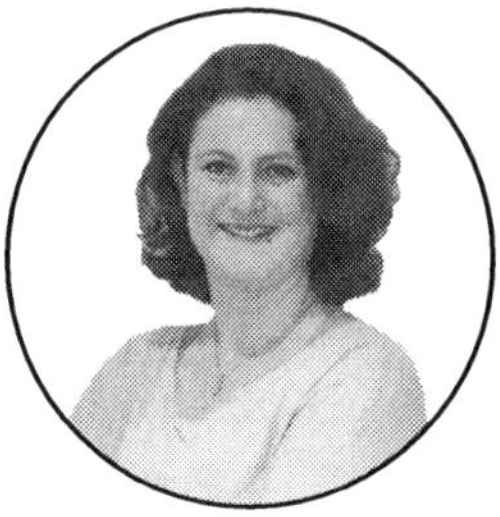

Beth is based in Limehouse, East London, where she lives with her partner and her much loved cat Lola. She loves flowers, live music and theatre and - having spent many years working in the investigation arena - is an avid watcher of crime dramas and thrillers and likes reading them too.

Having had to deal with her own back pain from a young age, her biggest passion is helping people get out of pain and move more freely and she says her investigation background definitely comes in handy when getting to the bottom of client's pain.

Beth, who is an award-winning business owner, has a fully equipped Pilates and movement therapy studio in Limehouse and also works with clients virtually.

Website: www.bethredfernpilates.co.uk

Email: beth@bethredfernpilates.co.uk

Back Pain - An Integrated Approach Looking At The Whole Picture

When and where did you first experience back pain? For me it was in my early teens when I couldn't join in the fun on a family day out because my back was hurting. At 16 I was diagnosed with a disease in my spine (after I couldn't stand up at the end of one of my school exams, which was pretty scary for my teenage self) and from then on suffered periodic bouts of back pain that would sometimes get so bad I'd be unable to move. Then, at 25, I found myself in hospital having emergency back surgery. Unfortunately, surgery didn't stop the pain and over the next few years (when again once or twice a year I'd be immobile) I felt like my back ruled my life and tried lots of different things to find a solution, including swimming, prescription painkillers, a hospital run pain management course, several epidural injections into my spine and seeing a variety of different practitioners who, although some were fantastic and helped me move forward, were never able to provide a complete and longstanding solution to my pain. After one particular flare up things got so bad that for several years during my late 30s I could hardly function and my quality of life was miserable.

That was before the approach I'm going to talk about in this chapter helped me take back control.

It changed everything for me, not just physically in terms of reducing my pain, improving my mobility and rebuilding my confidence in my back so I could do the things I loved, but mentally and emotionally too. Would you like to take back some control? If I can do it, you can too!

I'd read about Pilates being good for back care and, having joined a local class, fell in love with it. I learnt exercises I could do at home to look after myself and, in taking back some control, found I no longer panicked when I could feel my back getting worse. This was amazing! However, when I had flare ups I couldn't go to my class so began private lessons on the specialist Pilates equipment which always helped me, no matter how I was feeling. This impacted me so profoundly that I decided to train as a teacher and subsequently left my 20 year career with one of the 'Big 4' accountancy firms to follow my passion. Since then, in my quest to provide the best for my clients (many of whom are professional women much like I was), I've explored other therapies that complement the Pilates work that I do, testing them out on my own body before training in them so I know they really work. Clinical biomechanics, massage, mindfulness, myofascial release and yoga inspired movement are now integral to my practice. Working in a fully integrated way has been game changing both for my own body and for how I now work with my clients, allowing me to 'problem solve' and approach their issues from lots of different angles to get the best results.

This unique and seamlessly integrated approach which has been so life changing for me (I now feel and move better than I have for the last 20 years) has had a huge impact on many of my clients. For instance, I was recently referred a client who, having tried a number of other treatment and exercise options as well as being on strong prescription medication, came to see me for help with what she described as 'severe' back pain from a bulging disc which she said was getting worse. By the end of our first session her pain had reduced significantly and when I saw her four days later she told me that she'd been able to stop taking her pain medication and that her chiropractor (who she'd seen the previous day) wanted to speak to me because he was so amazed at the change in her.

In addition, another client came to see me having been suffering with back pain for which he'd seen several different medical specialists over the previous three months. Having conducted my usual in-depth assessment (after which this client told me I'd given him more information than any of the medical specialists had) I gave him two very simple exercises to do daily at home. A week later he told me his pain had significantly reduced and within only a few weeks it had completely gone. Having checked with both of these clients for permission to use their stories, I can confirm that they are both still pain free. I also recently worked with a lady with upper back, neck and shoulder pain who told me after only two weeks of working with me that she felt better than she'd ever felt in her whole adult life.

If - like I used to be - you're fed up of having to rely on others to keep you functioning (so you can carry on working, looking after your family and having some kind of a life), you're tired of seeing different practitioners but nothing seems to work long term, you've had enough of finding everyday tasks difficult and missing out on fun or your hobbies, or you feel like your back rules your life (or certainly defines your day), here are some of the key lessons I've learnt from the last 35 plus years of managing my own back condition, as well as working with my clients:

- Make sure that whoever you work with (whether a hands on practitioner or a movement professional) addresses your whole body and looks for what's causing the pain or problem rather than just focusing on the area that hurts and dealing with your symptoms. Where pain is experienced isn't necessarily where the problem started so looking at the whole body for the root cause is paramount. If they don't find the root cause, then even if they get you out of pain, it's likely to come back again, and ideally you want them to stop the problem from happening again.
- Be proactive about managing your condition so that you're a part of the solution rather than simply relying on others to 'fix' you. Not only will you benefit physically, but you'll feel so much more empowered and in control. When you're in pain it can be scary to move, but unless you've been told by your medical practitioner that you shouldn't, movement will usually help and if you're seeing a practitioner, a good Pilates practice will help your body maintain the adjustments they've made so that you feel the benefit longer term. In my experience the clients who get the best results are the ones who do their homework, so if you're given exercises to do at home, do them and do them regularly (if you find this hard, work with someone who'll give you support and accountability)! If you're

nervous about moving, or you want to learn the best way to use exercise to help you, find a good movement teacher who you resonate with and who is confident with back pain. In dealing with my own pain over the years, I was most successful when working with someone I trusted and who I felt understood what I was going through and I've been told by many clients that this is one of the things they value about working with me.

- Consider how your lifestyle, posture, movements and habits may be impacting you - when I work with clients it's not just about the time they spend with me, but what they do the rest of the week that we work on. Developing whole body awareness is crucial (which is why it's so central to my integrated approach). How is your body positioned when you sit, stand and walk? How do you move between sitting and standing, lying and sitting (some of my clients have felt significant reductions in pain simply by learning better strategies for these everyday movements)? Are you using your lower back to make movements that should be made at your hips? Are your feet and ankles stiff (I love barefoot shoes by the way)? Do you change positions regularly? Lie ins are lovely, but if you feel stiff in the mornings could getting up earlier help? Do you pace your activities so that you don't let your pain build up?

If you'd like to find out more about my integrated approach you can get in touch on beth@bethredfernpilates.co.uk or head over to my website www.bethredfernpilates.co.uk where you can book an in person or virtual Discovery session.

Simon Rogers

The Feel Better Coach

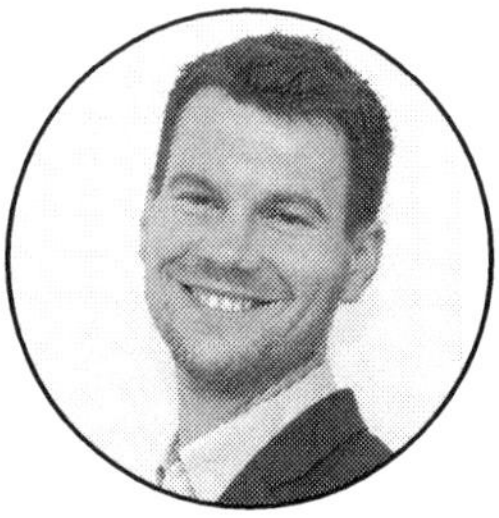

Simon has worked with thousands of clients across Europe for over 15 years. He has helped them solve long-standing stress-related upper back and neck pain leading them to live more successful and fulfi lling lives.

He's found that working with people as people, physically, emotional and mentally rather than focusing only on their symptoms allows them to work at the root cause. This provides them with not only a lasting solution to their pain but means that they can fall in love with a life that they are now consciously creating.

What would you be able to do if you were able to solve your pain for good?

Website: www.restoreyourbodynow.co.uk

Email: simon@restoreyourbodynow.co.uk

Phone: +44(0)2083 966 668

Pain That Doesn't Come Back

Close your eyes, now imagine you waved a magic wand and your back pain disappeared? It was just gone! And now you could also trust your back to keep up with you in whatever you wanted to do. That same pain back that pestered you with an annoying ache, whispered to you that you needed to reign yourself in and not be too ambitious. It distracted you worried that it might give way just when wanted to pick up your child or grandchild. It made you miss the moment. It made you feel that you could live your life the way you wanted, the way that you knew would be possible if that damn pain was gone for good! So how do you feel now that you have waved your magic wand and it has disappeared for good?

Many of my clients have experienced what it's like to suffer from long-term back pain only for them to experience freedom from it and start to live their lives in a way that they had almost given up on. Take for example Grace, a middle-aged mother to a teenage daughter and busy postal worker. When I first met Grace, she had had back pain and knee pain for more than a decade. Grace opened up about how much life was increasingly becoming a burden to her due to her physical and emotional discomfort. Grace was being supported by her GP and had been using a high dosage of anti-depressants for over 20 years. We started working together and within a couple of months Grace was having far less pain in her back and knee. She was also amazed that she also felt so much better inside! Grace excitedly shared that she was going to have a conversation with her GP to plan to come off of her anti-depressants all together. Grace is now trusting her back and knee and is feeling better than she can ever remember. She has changed not only her back and knee pain for good but also her whole outlook on her future!

I've worked with thousands of clients like Grace that were seeking a solution to their long-term back pain. Through my experience I've developed a unique 3-step system that I use to support every client through their journey from limiting back pain to freedom from it. And I'm going share it with you right now! My 3-step system is: **Identify**, **Resolve**, **Create.** What Does that mean? Well, **Identify** the root cause of your pain, **Resolve** the problems in your body that lead to your pain, then **Create** the life you really want to have now that you are not limited by pain.

Working with many clients has led me to notice some common mistakes that so many make and that have got in the way of them solving their back pain for good. These are the insights that I share with every client so that they get better results and can get back to enjoying their lives. Would you like me to share these mistakes that, if you are making them too, are seriously getting in your way? I'm assuming that was a resounding yes!

Here are the 3 mistakes:

1. We misunderstand what the problem actually is.
2. We treat our bodies as if they were machines.

3. We believe that pain = damage!

None of these are true!

In place of these common mistakes, I help my clients to understand that:

1. Our symptoms are not the problem. We need to identify the actual problem and root cause of it.

2. Our bodies have an innate healing ability and it is important to trust in this!

3. Pain = attention please! We need to listen to understand the messages from our bodies.

There's a cartoon image I often describe to my clients to show them what I mean by 'our symptoms are not the problem'. It shows two men frantically mopping up a flooded bathroom floor. When you look in the background of the image, you can see that a basin is overflowing with water and the tap is still running. This is what I see initially that my clients don't yet see. Your pain, the symptom, is definitely a problem! I get that and, from my expert view, I understand what is happening in your body that is leading to the pain being there. So, pain isn't THE problem. If it was the problem, I'm sure you would have solved it yourself. That's part of the reason we go to an expert for a solution, because you can't identify the problem yourself. Not only do we want to identify the problem but also the causes of it to ensure that this problem stays resolved long-term. This mean we must identify the root cause.

I often find that my clients treat their bodies as if they were machines. If its broken, then it needs fixing or parts need replacing. What is missing is the understanding that our body has an amazing ability to heal itself! When we cut our finger, it heals with no intervention from us other than possibly a plaster. It would be amazing if your car would do the same, right?! We need to learn to trust in the innate healing ability more and instead ask the question what might we be doing that is impeding this and how can we best assist our body to heal itself?

I find that many of my clients also misunderstand pain and it's no surprise why. Pain is a complex process. For practical use the assumption that pain = damage is in many cases not only inaccurate but unhelpful. When you believe that pain = damage, it gets in the way of your body's healing ability. Essentially, we have two modes that manage our bodily functions; 1. Sympathetic - fight, fright, flight or 2. Parasympathetic – rest, digest, heal. These modes function like a seesaw where, when the activity of one mode is increased, the other is decreased. When we believe something is broken or damaged, we tend to stress about it and therefore the sympathetic activity is increased. This means that parasympathetic activity is decreased, so your body is less able to rest, digest and heal. This is the power of a story that you believe in! A more useful perspective is pain = attention please! With this attention we need to listen to understand the messages from our body. The pain is there is to remind you that there is still a problem and causes of this problem leading to the pain. It's reminding you to find a solution to the problem.

My hope is that reading this has given you the hope that you can not only get relief from your back pain, you can have freedom from it for good!

If you are curious about what is possible for you or a loved one, then I have a special gift for you. If you send 'Solve my back pain for good' to hello@restoreyourbodynow.co.uk then I will send you a complimentary video series to get you started on your journey.

Mark Roughley

Expert in lower back pain relief

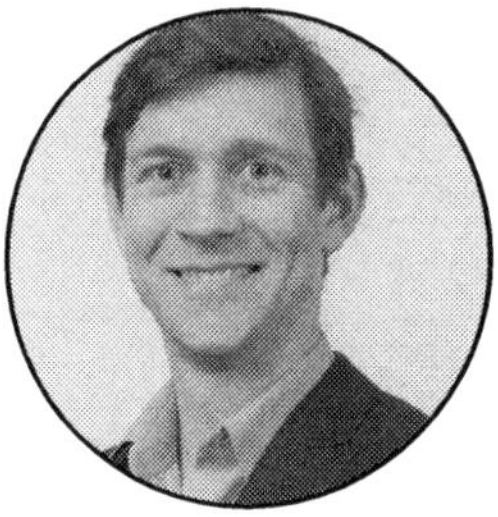

With a background in engineering and 11 years of experience working as a top osteopath, Mark is an expert at helping people suffering with lower back pain. He has worked all over the world and helped thousands of people recover from the most debilitating lower back conditions.

He is a firm believer in helping patients to help themselves and is passionate about the overall health and wellbeing of his patients. He loves the experience of working with clients to restore their quality of life and happiness, assisting them to move forwards leaving the lower back pain a distant memory.

He loves running, wrestling with his children and dreams of fulfilling a lifelong ambition of having a pet pig.

Website: www.osteopathiccentre.co.uk

Email: enquiries@leominsterosteopaths.co.uk

Phone: +44(0)1568 610 610

Did You Know That Lower Back Pain (LBP) Affects Up To 80% Of The Adult Population Of The UK At Least Once During Their Lives?

What if I told you that with a little understanding you could minimise your risk of getting it? Or if I could tell you how best to manage it at home if you do develop it?

A large proportion of that 80% can experience LBP several times throughout their lives and unfortunately for some, it can plague them continually for years. I've been in practice as an osteopath for 11 years and I've treated thousands of people with LBP. Over that time I've developed my own unique system to help my clients get the best outcome with treatment and to support home management.

I have found the keys to treating and managing LBP are:

- understanding why it happens
- a simple strategy to help recovery at home
- and how to minimise the risks of getting it or have it reoccur.

To understand why LBP happens we need to understand how the body works, moves and how it can be influenced. The first thing to try and picture is a human skeleton. The skeleton is the basic structure of the body; it provides protection for the organs by the hard bones and flexibility by the multitude of joints. The joints are held together by ligaments and moved by the muscles. Everything is attached to the bones of the skeleton and so everything relies on the bones being in their optimal position. The ideal position of the skeleton, or posture, is one that is symmetrical and balanced. If the skeleton loses an element of symmetry then the body has to work harder to maintain its upright position-try walking around leaning to the left; it becomes hard work after a while! The more out of kilter the skeleton is, the harder the body has to work to perform normal tasks. That extra stress is taken up the muscles, ligaments and spinal discs and once the stress eventually overloads the tissue, it will cause pain.

There are many factors that ultimately affect our posture:

- the type of work that we do (PC work, tradespeople, driving, farming)
- our pastimes (sports, gym, walking, gardening, travelling)
- what we do in our free time (watching TV, reading, socialising, gaming, checking phones)
- injuries we may have accrued (sports injuries, car crashes, falls)

All of these and many more things will affect how our posture develops over time. The single biggest influencer on our posture however is gravity. Gravity is a constant perpetual force that pulls us into the ground and our body's natural stance is to be upright. To stand tall our bodies have to battle the influence of gravity. Why does LBP occur so often? In my opinion it is because there is considerable weight bearing down on the lower back. It supports the abdomen in front and the chest, head, neck and arms above. It sits just above the pelvis and legs which give us the ability to walk. So the lower back has to be strong enough to support the body above and also be flexible enough to allow movement from the legs to transfer up the body. This is why it is more susceptible to injury than anywhere else in the body. We feel pain when something in the body is damaged. That can either come about from a trauma or develop over a long period of time. The vast majority of LBP cases I've seen have come seemingly out of nowhere but have, in reality, been building over many years. The posture will have become more and more misaligned and eventually the body can no longer cope with the strain. Something has to give, resulting in pain in the muscles, ligaments and spinal discs.

Any structure in the lower back can emit pain, however the what is not nearly as important as the why. The why comes from understanding what has happened before the pain has arisen, addressing this is how to get a long term solution rather than quick fix relief. Once the history behind the lower back pain has been understood, we can set about examining and treating the postural imbalances with hands on treatment. The whole skeleton is affected by postural changes, so when we experience LBP, I have found it's best to treat the whole body. This will positively affect the posture, encourage the body to heal, relieve pain and make long lasting changes.

If you suffer with LBP and you can't get to see someone about it you can still help yourself at home.

In my experience of treating thousands of people with LBP, the best thing to do is to rest. It's important to understand the healing process in the body is most effective when we are not physically doing anything. This does not mean lounging on the sofa, however. The most effective resting position is to lie on your back on the floor with several pillows or cushions under the back of the knees, with a cushion under the head for comfort. The legs should be relaxed, their weight supported by the cushions underneath so that there is an angle at the knees, allowing the base of the spine to relax. The best angle is different for different people but in general the knee angle shouldn't be greater than approximately 45 degrees. If the lower back is very painful or mobility is quite badly affected then try the same position on a bed, preferably a firm mattress. If in a lot of pain then resting like this 3 to 4 times a day for half an hour at a time is very helpful for getting pain relief, taking weight off the spine, and giving the body time to rest and heal. For less severe pain then swap sitting on the sofa to watch TV in an evening, with having a spell on the floor instead.

The best approach is to minimise the risk of getting LBP or have it return. Unfortunately there isn't a golden set of exercises to do each day, or a specific type of exercise that will protect us. I am often asked which is better yoga or Pilates; both have merits but I've also treated teachers of both disciplines for LBP. The answer lies in how we approach everything, making good habits, looking after our bodies and having awareness of our posture when we are performing tasks.

Here are a couple of examples of when making small adjustments had big results . Firstly, I was treating an elderly gentleman with long term lower backache;

after a few sessions of slow progress it transpired that he regularly chopped wood at the end of his garden and carried it 50 or so metres back to the house. I asked if he had a wheelbarrow and he confirmed he did and once he started to use that his recovery quickened and he was soon pain free. Secondly, a lady suffering with acute lower back pain would sit for a couple of hours a day in her favourite chair. It was positioned diagonally opposite her TV, and she would tuck her knees under her, twisting slightly in the chair. By moving her chair to be in line with the TV she didn't need to sit and twist in her seat and she also made a full recovery.

As described in the beginning most injuries are due to the cumulative effects of gravity, time and activities done poorly. We can't do anything about time or gravity but we can control how we do things such as

- sit in more supportive chairs,
- bend the knees when picking anything up whether it's a pencil or a brick,
- have regular coaching to improve how well we play our chosen sports,
- don't try to carry too much in one go
- use tools appropriately

These are very general ideas but they have to be because we all do so many different tasks throughout the day and throughout our lives. We can all improve on how we do things to help look after our lower backs now and for the future.

If you would like to know more about how I can help resolve your LBP then email enquiries@leominsterosteopaths.co.uk for a free assessment.

Karen Revivo

Physiotherapist Specialising in Upledger Craniosacral therapy

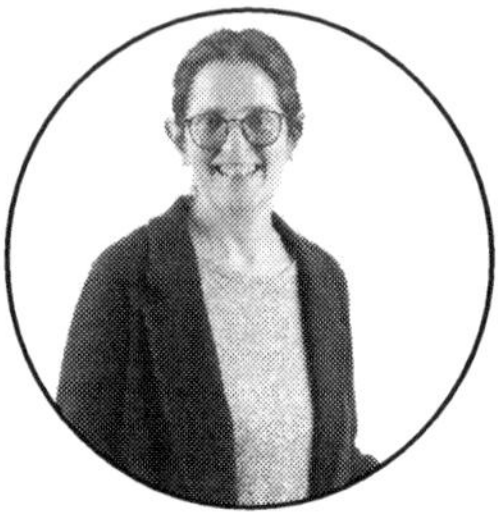

I help women reconnect with their bodies, get to the root of the problem and rebuild their trust in themselves.

Karen Revivo has over 35 years of experience in getting to the root cause of the presented problem. In recognising the complete interconnection of our mental,emotional and physical being. She has uniquely combined all of this into a system of working which is highly successful.

Working as a team with the client is important to Karen and so in 2011 she opened the Therapy Life Centre, a holistic centre integrating all the aspects of health needed to support her clients and their families.

Website: www.therapylifecentre.co.uk

Email: karenrevivo@therapylifecentre.co.uk

Phone: +44(0)7482 119 113

Death And Dental Work Caused My Back Pain? Connecting Unexpected Dots Between Your Life Experiences And Back Pain

When I was 11, my father died and when I was 21 I had four wisdom teeth removed. "What's the relevance of that?" I hear you ask. This is a book about back pain. It turns out, as I have discovered over my 36-year career, that these two events were catalysts of the long-term and consistent physical pain that I would experience. Back pain, neck pain and chronic headaches.

The problems didn't really start until a few weeks after having my wisdom teeth removed when I started experiencing severe lower back pains. It had started out of the blue and although I managed to keep the intrusive pain at bay it never went away. Roll on 20 years and things had deteriorated to the point where I had either lower back pain, neck pain or chronic headaches and often all 3. This was having a devastating impact on my life. I was struggling to have the energy to work and be the Mum I wanted to be to my two beautiful children. I had to choose between pain or that horrible feeling mothers get of letting their children down. Have you ever felt that? That constant battle of managing a chronic problem and juggling your own health needs with those of your family? Having to deal with the emotional impact that has on you?

I was seeing the same situation with my clients, pain being managed rather than cleared, watching the frustration but also the acceptance. That sense of 'Oh well, nothing I can do, I am stuck with it'. So now I was feeling that I was letting my clients down, as well as myself, and most importantly my family.

I recognised the mind-body connection and so I began to search for answers. The beginning of my own personal healing journey and that of hundreds of clients started when I went along to a workshop and had my mind totally blown. I was being treated by another attendee, the treatment took me back to a traumatic memory around my fathers' death that was locked inside of me. I was able to cry, process the memory and let it go. I then saw what was possible and the powerful results of working in this way.

Why do emotions have such an impact on our physical health? Emotions are an energy of sorts; when we suppress them, they get stuck. They create 'roadblocks' in our bodies, causing us to have to make diversions. Stuck emotions change the way we hold ourselves. By working with them through our physical body, we clear away the obstruction, allowing everything to flow again, helping our bodies to operate at their optimum levels.

Types of emotional problems are multiple. Trauma from childhood, a one-off major incident, or a dripping tap effect, in which small events build up and accumulate and create a block. Often, we are not even aware of the trauma and the impact it is having, as was the case with myself. I wonder if this has made you think of different experiences you have had in your life.

I remember a patient who was 25 when she came to see me with chronic lower back pain and severe issues with her periods. While I was working on her lower back, she suddenly experienced a spontaneous memory of being fifteen years old. While getting the bus home from school she had been standing by the driver waiting to get off, when the bus had hit and killed an elderly man. She had not told any friends or family and instead had locked it into her body. The dominant emotion that came from this memory was guilt, as she thought she had distracted the bus driver, causing the man's death. Through a process that we call Somatic Emotional Release (SER), we were able to connect with that 15-year-old girl and help her see what happened from a more mature perspective. This helped my patient to understand that it was not her fault, which was vital to her recovery. She had started her period the day that this event occurred; all the hidden trauma had become locked there, and as a result the physical discomfort of her periods was amplified to a level that made it extremely difficult. She had no idea that the two were connected. Once we were able to release the physical and emotional tension, she was free of back pain and notably, period pain.

Another formative experience occurred at a workshop which focused on the mouth and jaw. I was able to see what a traumatic tooth removal had done to my body. The top of my spine was jammed from the physical strain, the offset balance had a knock-on effect to my lower back, creating decades of pain. I had a new way of working with my clients, a way of understanding and relieving my own pain, which was truly liberating.

Would you believe you could clear low back pain by releasing the bones of the skull and jaw?

So let me tell you about one of my clients who was suffering from excruciating back and leg pain, for which he had seen doctors, had MRI scans, injections, and was facing the serious prospect of surgery. He could not move without being in agony, was unable to do his very physical job or play with his 6-year-old son. He came to see me after his wife had talked him into it; he didn't seem convinced; however he was running out of options. During the assessment, I learned that he had experienced head trauma as a youngster and had major root canal treatment two weeks before the onset of his pain. I explained to him how the two can be connected and so treated his jaw and skull, at no point did I touch his back. There was an immediate effect on his symptoms for the first time in three months. He was elated. Three sessions later, his pain had reduced dramatically. The last time I heard from him, he was back playing football with his son, thriving at work, and free of pain.

My patients and I are living testament to the fact that you can turn things around significantly by listening to and supporting the body to release all of these tensions whether they be emotional or physical.

I urge you to think outside the box when it comes to your health. Go back through your life and look at the different situations, physically and emotionally that have affected you. Then if you are curious to understand more about your own personal blocks please get in touch. Together we can explore what is in the way for you.

Adam Sealey

Based in Hertfordshire, Adam Sealey is one of the UK's leading back pain specialists

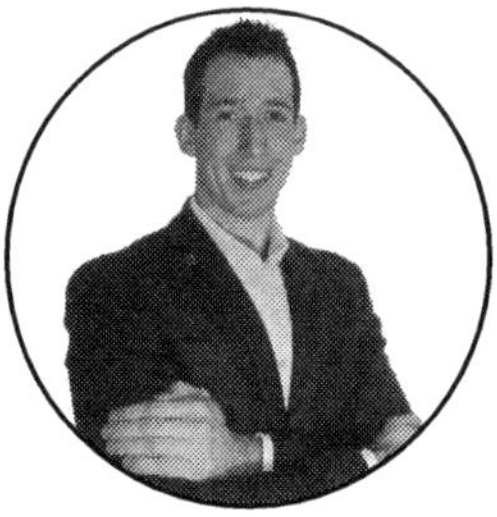

With almost a decade in the health and wellness industry, Adam specialises in working with those suffering with long term back pain and offers bespoke treatments that incorporate a variety of techniques.

From spinal manipulations to exercise prescription, Adam's unique treatment approach has successfully helped hundreds of his patients restore movement, improve function and ultimately rid them of their long term pain. These changes enable his patients to lead a lifestyle they never thought achievable.

Adam's passion and dedication for providing care to his patients has earned him a National Award from the Institute of Osteopathy as well as having his work published in Osteopathy Today Magazine and The Business Independent Magazine.

Website: www.backpainsolutions.co.uk

Email: adam@sealeyosteopathy.com

What If I Told You That You Can Permanently Resolve Your Long-Term Back Pain, No Matter How Many Years You've Had It For?

Would you believe me if I told you that I've successfully helped hundreds of clients resolve their back pain in just three easy steps? Sounds too good to be true, right? Wrong. I've developed these three steps to help my clients take back control and resolve their pain independently, instead of having to put their faith in a practitioner for potentially years of treatment. By the time you've finished reading this chapter, you'll know exactly how these three steps can work for you too.

Speaking of faith, who am I to be giving you this 'too good to be true' advice? Let me introduce myself:

My name is Adam Sealey and I'm an award winning back pain specialist based in Hertfordshire who has been working with clients with long-term back pain for close to a decade. Early on in my career, (as most manual therapists often do) I tried to help everyone that walked into my clinic regardless of their particular ailment. Such conditions often included Arthritis, Bunions, Carpal tunnel syndrome.....a literal ABC of medical problems. However, it was only after a few years of practice I truly began to appreciate how long-term pain tends to heal over a far longer timeframe.

I couldn't expect the same quick results as other conditions. Simply put, the longer you've had a bad back, the harder it is to resolve. This added difficulty drove me to develop my own unique approach that has helped hundreds of clients resolve their long-term back pain and I aim to teach you too.

To help illustrate my system, I'm going to introduce you to a client of mine called Mike. Mike is a single dad in his 40's who's been putting up with back pain for the best part of ten years. Mike works a typical 9-5 desk job and has noticed that over the last five years his back has noticeably deteriorated to the point where he is in day to day discomfort. The day Mike finally decided to book an appointment with me was the day he found he was in too much pain to play with his son.

Upon his arrival, one of the first steps Mike and I went through is what I like to call:

Speed Date Your Back!

In order to get a deeper understanding of what makes Mike's back pain tick, I asked him to approach the situation like he was speed dating - find out what his back likes and doesn't like!

I asked Mike to write down EVERYTHING he could think of that affects his back pain and organise it into two lists: 'likes' and 'dislikes.' Mike's list included things such as 'it hurts when I sit for long hours' and 'it feels better at the weekends.' There are no right or wrong answers.

Next, I asked Mike to imagine a set of scales where each item on his list corresponds to its own individual weight. On one side of the scale he stacked up everything that aggravated or prolonged his back pain and on the other side he stacked up the things that helped it.

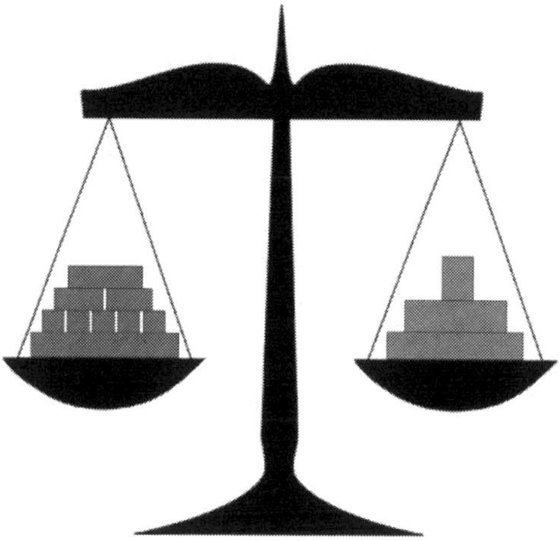

These imaginary weights varied in size depending on how much of an impact they had; Mike included a large weight in his 'likes' that represented an exercise for his back that he found to be beneficial. Unfortunately he had far more weights on the 'dislikes' side which meant that even though the stretch was beneficial, it simply wasn't enough to help. For Mike to see progress, we needed to tip the scales in favour of getting better by reducing the weight on the 'dislikes' side of the scale and increasing the weight on the 'likes' side.

What is your scale looking like? Is it balanced or uneven? Try to go through your list and add/remove as many as you can to help tip the scales towards positive change. The bigger the shift towards the 'likes' side then the faster your recovery will be.

Mike found that long hours sitting was the biggest contributor to his pain so he managed to get a standing desk. This single action made a huge difference to his recovery. You should also have a variety of actions that you can start implementing straight away.

Although Mike was excited to see progress, it came slowly. This however didn't come as a surprise and leads me nicely onto the next step:

Be a Good Patient by Being Patient!

As I mentioned earlier, long-term back pain by its very definition can take a long time to heal and you need to be in the right state of mind to prepare for a long journey. Expecting a quick fix will demoralise you and regularly leads people to the incorrect conclusion that it can't be fixed at all. How long exactly I can't say, but 9 times out of 10 it's going to take longer than you think. Unfortunately, long-term back pain tends to perpetuate itself until you give it a reason to begin healing. My role is to essentially strong-arm your healing mechanisms into action when they have long since given up. So trust me when I say you'll do yourself a massive favour by being patient – the results will be worth the wait!

So, Mike now has a daily list of actions and is mentally prepared for the process, but what else could he be doing outside of the treatment room?

Keep Active

The general rule is that the body likes to move; this is what it's designed for and a lot of healing processes require movement in order to work effectively.

Mike found swimming helped his back but he would only go once a month, so we upped it to twice weekly. If you find that you already have physical activities on your 'likes' list then just carry on with these. If you're not particularly active, then we can try to base the type of activity you do on the lists you've just completed. For Mike, his back felt better when he curled up into a ball, so I prescribed exercises that encouraged this movement such as hamstring stretches. Once you know what your own back prefers, you can try out stretches and exercises that cater to those positions. I'd always recommend starting with low intensity movements like those in yoga or Pilates and build up from there. This is one of those few times where Google can be your friend; a bit of time researching basic yoga or Pilates for beginners will generate lots of exercises. All you then need to do is cherry-pick the ones that compliment your 'likes' list.

Review

1. **Be a Good Patient by Being Patient!**
2. **Speed Date Your Back!**
3. **Keep Active**

Mike is now not only pain free but he's also more physically active, self-aware and most importantly he's able to be the type of father to his son that he wanted to be. It sounds almost *too* simple, but these steps have transformed Mike's life and they can transform yours too.

If you follow the steps and a few weeks pass with no sign of improvement, then I would suggest either revisiting your list or seeking out professional help. Sometimes even with the best will in the world, some things aren't able to make a full recovery without the help of a professional to identify crucial weaknesses or imbalances.

If this is the case or you are just concerned about your back pain then I am more than happy to discuss your situation. As a reader of this book you'll get a free consultation with me (valued at £75) where we can examine your back issues and explore your next step. If you happen to be local then this can be face to face, or part of my online service.

To organise your free consultation you can email adam@sealeyosteopathy.com, but please feel free to email me as I'd love to hear about your progress.

Gordon Sharp

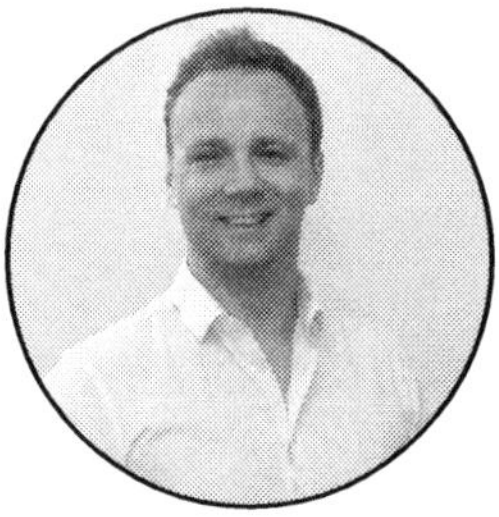

Gordon Sharp is the Head Therapist and Owner of Massage Weymouth who sees himself as a unique back specialist. Unique is a hard word to quantify - but with a background in Dance, experience in Life-coaching, Fitness instructing, full qualifications in Sort tissue Therapy and a childhood trauma that was potentially crippling – unique seems a fair word here.

His clientele ranges from Olympians and European Champions to Fund raisers and the general public in the street! He primarily works with the middle-aged, often with a sporting background who have been suffering for more than six weeks. It all adds up to an interesting story that Gordon would like to share with you.

Website: www.gordonsharp.com

Email: gordon@gordonsharp.com

Phone: +44(0)7894 709 904

What If Back Pain Was A Thing Of Your Past?

Said the man that couldn't walk & then became a professional dancer.

If you are reading this, chances are you either have a bad back, know someone with a bad back or want insight into bad backs. Let me share a secret with you... your bad back is special. It's unique. It's yours!

Talking of unique, what makes me such a unique back specialist?

It's not just about qualifications and experience. I believe that to become a specialist you have to gain an insight into your clients and their lives. They're a real person. I want to know their lifestyle and mindset. You need to get to know them as an individual so that you can treat them as an individual, otherwise you may never get to the root cause of their pain in the first place.

My name is Gordon and this is the story of how I became the specialist I am today. I am telling my story so that you can get to know me as a person, as well as a therapist, to find out in more detail how I work and whether my work and experience could help you. I will also offer some simple and effective tips to help you with back pain.

When I say my story starts at the very beginning, I mean it. Literally, within the first few moments of my life I was dropped on my back and head. This left me physically and mentally handicapped for those first few years of my life. Specialists from around the world said that I would *never* walk. Through the patient persistence of my parents, physiotherapists, massage specialists and (I like to think) my own determination, by the age of five I had defied their prognosis. There was, however, a legacy. My natural stance was to walk backwards, and my coordination was back to front, which made it very difficult to do the simplest of activities (apart from backwards races on Sports Day, which I always won!) When I started walking forwards a year later, one thing was drilled into me from every person involved in my care – *when you stand up, stand up straight*. Not like a regimented soldier, just stand up straight *before you start moving*. This engages the neural pathways so that your body and mind can connect and reduces pressure on the back.

The lesson here is to *be patient with yourself.* Performing this simple exercise - standing up straight before you start - can get you moving better. *Posture is key to improving back pain.*

At six I decided I wanted to dance. With my weight not neutrally positioned and my back arching a lot, I had to be trained to have strong core stability and my balance to be neutral or leant forward. This was the complete opposite to what was natural to me. However, after years of training, I managed to become a professional dancer and continued for sixteen years. Dancing teaches you how your body works and how you compensate for the pressures that you place upon it. Your back needs core stability to support it. Core stability isn't just about stomach muscles - it requires strength from your hamstrings right up to the lower thoracic parts of your spine. You need to concentrate on all of these muscles, with all of the origins and insertions, to make sure that you get a strong, reliable back. If one of these muscle groups are tight or weak, then that will automatically affect your back mobility and posture. If improving core stability resonates with you, contact me and I will gladly guide you through the appropriate information for you. After all, your back is unique.

As a professional dancer you learn how to read your dance partner and the people that you work with, as quickly as you can. The simplest look or movement of their body can tell you if that person is feeling safe, steady or unsure. This became second nature and I use that intuition in every treatment I do, so I can quickly start a treatment that is **specifically tailored to the clients individual needs**. You also need to discover if you are the right therapist for that person.

Today, I primarily work with men aged 45 to 55 from a sporting background, who have been suffering from lower back pain for more than six weeks. I get them onto the right path to recovery and becoming pain free, allowing them to achieve their goals as well as feeling comfortable and more confident in everyday life.

Within a year of qualifying as a therapist (supported by my dancers knowledge and the additional qualifications of being a fitness instructor and NLP – Life Coach) I started working with some of the top Olympians in the world. This work continued for four years, taking me around the UK and Europe.

The Australian Olympic Sailing Team said:

"He listens to each person and individualises their treatment, to ensure their needs are being met." Have I mentioned / highlighted that already? They also said, *"His knowledge and skills have proven to be of a high level."*

While working with the elite I was also building up a client base in my hometown. I had the pleasure of treating Ben, who wanted to inspire children and raise public awareness of bullying. He completed 401 marathons in 401 days and formed the "401 Challenge Foundation Charity" which gained him a highly prestigious award. After helping Ben, his testimonial said, *"I met a lot of therapists throughout my journey around the UK and I can categorically say that Gordon was one of the best"*.

We're not all Athletes or Olympians though and we all have different goals. Goals depend on where you currently are in life, from running your next marathon to walking to the shops – without pain. Having regular treatments and an individualised self-care routine actually works out more beneficial than injuries hindering your income and achievements.

Giles (a GBR European Champion Triathlete in his age group) knows first-hand the importance of having regular treatments with the right therapist, to enable him to compete in international events and achieve his goals. Giles said, *"I could not perform to the best of my ability without him (Gordon)."*

Rome wasn't built in a day. No-one can wave a magic wand – improvement requires patience. Unless you make changes to the way that you do things, such as posture and technique, you will keep coming back to the same fundamental problems. You need to address the underlying causes, not just the symptoms, which requires one to be aware of strengths and weaknesses (not 'over-doing it', as an example).

Now you know why your posture, core stability and patience are key to having a healthy back. There are simple exercises you can do at home without any equipment. If any pain occurs stop immediately and seek specialist advice. Remember to build up the time on each exercise slowly - aim for one minute on each exercise to start with. Building the muscles gradually will also build your confidence, which will help improve posture.

A Daily Posture check.

1. Stand with the back of your head against a wall. Place your heels six inches from the wall. Your shoulder blades and butt should be touching the wall too.

2. There should be less than 2 inches between both your neck and the wall and your back and the wall. A larger gap indicates weak posture and a curving spine.

The recommended exercises below (and more) will help. Contact me and I will guide you through them via video link and personal free advice by telephone.

Child's Pose - Lengthens and stretches the spine, which is prone to slouching.

Cat-Cow - Activates the back and core muscles and helps increase an awareness of your back in relation to the rest of your body. If you feel uncomfortable on hands and knees, the Standing Cat-Cow is an alternative.

Remember, your bad back is special. Let me help you get onto the right pathway to recovery.

Stay safe and achieve your goals, Gordon Sharp

Head Therapist and Owner of Massage Weymouth

Graham Stones

Making you the hero of your pain journey

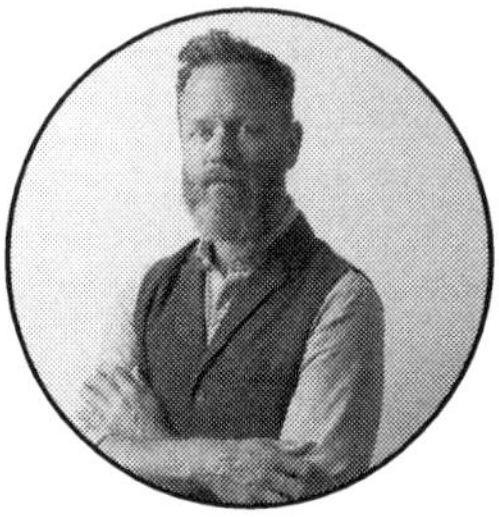

When you've fought back from near-certain death, you know that anything you want to achieve is possible. In December 2004, as a tsunami tore through South East Asia, Graham Stones was pulled underwater, his leg trapped between two tree trunks. With moments left to live, his leg freed itself and he, unlike many others, survived. But Graham was left with significant emotional and physical trauma.

The position of vulnerability he found himself in was new to Graham, a black belt in Kung Fu and dedicated yogi. Living in constant pain - a daily reminder of his trauma - Graham researched and practiced underutilised but proven recovery practices that could connect the missing links to pain free movement.

His path to recovery has since informed his blended approach which looks beyond treating just the muscles and joints to also treat the deeper internal structures of the body: the organs, nerves and fascia, often ignored in more conventional practices.

Because of his personal experience, Graham understands that pain is not just physical, and he is passionate about supporting people to return to their fullest, most joyful lives.

Over two decades Graham has been using a broad range of physical therapies and has a proven track record of achieving spectacular results, particularly for those struggling with long term back pain who feel like they have tried everything. His services have been employed by the English National Ballet and, as founder of Pain Free Movement ltd, by thousands of people looking to defeat pain, turn back the clock on their body and enjoy pain free movement again.

Website: www.painfree-movement.com

Email: freedom@painfree-movement.com

Phone: +44(0)7901 975 007

Pain Has Been Tricking You Into Asking The Wrong Question For Years!

By changing just one word you could discover a proven pathway to pain free movement.

Graham Stones applies his three-step pain free movement system to turn the nagging question of 'what is it?' to '*that* is it!' and helps his clients become the heroes of their pain journey.

When a prominent dancer from the English National Ballet was referred to me recently with crippling back pain, I knew the stakes were high. His entire livelihood rested on the health of his body, and it was broken. He was starting to panic after seeing different physicians and being given conflicting advice, none of which had improved his outcome. But I do things differently. Pain affects all aspects of your life: work, relationships, confidence; it can also lead to anxiety, or even depression. I know, because I've been there.

In 2004 I had a thriving sports therapy business, practicing conventional therapies. I was successful because I was talented at working painful areas and providing great relief - albeit temporary. But that year, my life changed forever, as well as my understanding of pain.

On Boxing Day 2004 I was in South East Asia when a tsunami tore through the coastlands. I was consumed by a wave and submerged, my leg trapped between two trees. I fought to release it, until I gave in, committing myself to the inevitable. As my body relaxed, my leg freed itself and I was able to swim to the surface and gain refuge on a rooftop. I had survived not by fighting, but by releasing tension. I was a fortunate survivor, but in the following years I battled with chronic pain, a constant reminder of what I'd been through and a source of anxiety. I felt crippled and aged, and the conventional methods I was turning to for relief were falling short. I wasn't ready to give up, and so I researched and started to practice proven, but underutilised methods. It worked.

Many of my clients have had similar experiences with pain: seeing practitioner after practitioner and never seeing results, or at best, temporary relief. I realised that this is not enough. When your pain is a crippling axe waiting to fall at any moment, how can you live a life with freedom and without fear? When pain causes you to feel helpless and older than your years, permanent change has to be the goal.

My personal experience taught me that pain is not the problem; it's your body's way of communicating the problem. But it can be deceptive. If all we do is treat the immediate source of pain, without looking into its cause, there can be no long-term relief. I specialise in helping clients to identify the root of the pain, turning "What is it?" into "THAT is it!" It's a really empowering moment in my clients' journey, to finally understand what is causing the pain they have been experiencing, some for many years. When they understand that they can not only relieve the pain, they can take back control and transform from pain victim to victor it is a revelation.

In my work I apply my pioneering three-step system to get to the source and turn back the clock on pain, to help you regain control, allowing you to move, own and use your body again. To do this I apply an understanding of how our complex internal systems work and their effect on the muscles and joints. The body is not made of separate elements, they are all interweaved and can all shift, creating a domino effect of different outcomes. When there is a problem with an organ, for example, your body will prioritise support to that area, affecting not only adjoining and connected tissues, but support systems elsewhere.

Unlocking the body's protective mechanisms releases tight, painful muscles and joints easily. When someone is in pain, they often believe that they need to crack or click away the pain but only to have it come back again. What I have discovered over the last twenty years is that it doesn't matter how good the manipulation is if it is not where your body is really saying the problem is then it will have little long term effect. The key is in the question "What is it?" When I help my clients figure out how to turn their nagging "what is it" into a specific "that is it!" it creates a powerful unlocking of tension for them. As the body relaxes, the spine begins to move easily and without tension or strain. But there is another advantage. As the treatments improve overall body function, clients report that their digestion is improved, they can sleep better, have more energy and feel better than they have in years. The treatment helps clients regain their lives and many report they feel younger than they have in years.

In my clinic I've seen thousands of clients who have been struggling with the nagging question of "what is it?", who need to regain movement and reclaim their sense of self. With my treatment I've seen them progress through their pain and come out the other end feeling like heroes: stronger, fitter and more confident than ever. I work with people from all backgrounds, but specialise in working with people who are struggling to find a solution to long term back pain. I thrive off helping them regain their freedom of movement and often their livelihoods, which are such a huge part of their identity.

I'm privileged to have been a part of the English National Ballet's medical team for the last 12 years and supported many of their dancers, including our earlier-mentioned friend. He had come to me close to desperation with a slipped disc. His successful career was on the line at a time when he had landed an important upcoming role. I knew I had to work quickly and effectively. Instead of treating the slipped disc I searched for and located the real source of pain and he gradually gained more release in his back and hip. A month later he messaged me to say that he felt like a new man, awakened from the fog of pain and better than he had in years. He was working as hard as ever, pain free.

An actor I worked with who had a slipped disc in his lower back told me that he wasn't really sure what I was doing or how but he knew that it was working. His spine specialist was shocked to see his progress, informing him that recovery from a spinal protrusion tends to take anywhere from 12 to 18 months. He was able to return to his acting work after just six months. This is what I live for. This is my passion.

When you live in constant pain, and especially if you have for years, it's easy to fall into a belief that this is what your life will be forever. But for many people, there can be real, permanent change. They can take charge of their pain and banish it for good.

Head on over to www.painfree-movement.com to see how I can help you today.

Congratulations!

Now you've reached the end of the book, the action starts. Depending on how you have read this book, now might be the time to go back and take some notes or even re-read a couple of chapters.

What are your key learnings from what you've read?

What are the top 5 things that you can perhaps change, tweak or add into your life to make a difference based on what you have read? Take the time to write these down as the act of writing will help cement them in your mind.

1.

2.

3.

4.

5.

Reading is of course valuable, yet it's taking action on what we've learned that creates change in our lives. Change can be both scary and exciting because it means doing things differently and creating a different and perhaps unknown outcome. With what you've learned from this book and the actions you're now going to take, what might now be possible for you, your family or loved ones?

Often, we look at the negatives of change and keep ourselves stuck because it feels safer.

We would challenge you to look at the positives

of change and get yourself moving physically or metaphorically. List out 5 great things that might be possible for you if you started adopting some of the suggestions from this book:

1.

2.

3.

4.

5.

By the way, if you found it challenging fill in this list, perhaps going back and re-reading or studying some of the chapters could help you get clear on what could become possible for you now.

However, if you're struggling with the idea of re-reading a book or 'studying' it then perhaps this example might help. As a Bikram yoga devotee, Karene used to do the same 26 postures in every Bikram yoga class and she used to do 1 or 2 classes every day. Yet every time, each class was different because she was different. Perhaps she had slept differently, or had different experiences meaning she had more or less energy to bring to class. Some days her favourite posture turned out to be the one she struggled with the most; or the one posture she didn't usually like became the one that made a real difference to her mood that day! It is same with books....there is always something new to 'see' when we re-read something because each time we read it, we are different. We have a different mindset and different emotions because we've had different experiences since we last read the book.

This means we are going to notice and remember different things when we re-read it.

So, by all means if you have enjoyed this book, pass it on to a friend, colleague or loved one and also revisit and re-read it for the lessons, stories and possibilities it might provide for you in the future. We know that not all of the authors, stories or experiences will resonate with you first time round and yet others may be the start of a new journey for you. We encourage you to reach out personally to those authors who 'spoke' to you to see what else they might be able to offer as support on your journey or just to feed back the difference their words have made for you.

We all go through life as individuals, however, it is the experience of relating to other humans where the magic happens. When we relate to others, we learn more about ourselves. We hope that this book has allowed you to 'meet' some more people and gain a deeper understanding of yourself.

We, and the authors who have made this possible, wish you every success with your journey.

Best wishes

Chris, Karene & David

About The Authors & HCB Publishing

David Gil Cristobal turns people into brands so they earn what they are worth and conquer the box seat in their customer's head. With more than three decades experience in the sports and business arena, David had a long career as a professional soccer player, before co-founding Eerion Performance, one of Switzerland's top health and fitness organisations, and launching Fitness Fortune University where he turns health and fitness professionals into elite fitness businesses in as little as 90 days. His clients typically increase their income by $50,000-100,000 within 12 months of implementing his systems. He has personally trained more than 1000 company teams in how to scale their businesses to new levels and experts in how to build 6 figure businesses.

Armed with a masters degree in business management and leadership, having built multiple 5, 6, and 7 figure businesses of his own, spoken to more than 100,000 people at Business and Financial conferences around the world in 13 different countries on 3 different continents, meeting business authorities and opinion leaders such as Sir Richard Branson, Tony Robbins, Kevin Harrington, Kane & Alessia Minkus and Herman Scherer, best-selling author off 5 books in 2 different languages, David speaks 6 languages, and has starred in a motion picture.

Chris and Karene Lambert-Gorwyn are the founders of Heart Centred Business Ltd and the authors of the #1 Amazon Best-Selling Book, Grow Your Heart Centred

Business from Passion to Profit. Having built multiple 5, 6 and 7 figure businesses of their own, Chris & Karene have been humbled with numerous Business Awards. They've spoken at Business and Financial conferences around the world in 14 different countries on 4 different continents, meeting business titans such as Sir Richard Branson, Les Brown, Tony Robbins, Randi Zuckerberg, Kevin Harrington, Gill Fielding, Nick James, Kane & Alessia Minkus and Robert & Kim Kiyosaki.

Chris & Karene grow Heart Centred Businesses and their clients typically increase their income by £50,000-100,000 within 12 months of implementing their systems. Teaching the right things in the right order, Chris & Karene have personally trained more than 3000 practitioners and experts how to build 6 figure businesses.

HCB Publishing

Chris, Karene and David founded HCB Publishing to help more business owners share their expertise with the world Do you have a special skill or expertise? Would you be curious to know how to use books to exponentially grow your business?

If you want to talk further and get direct support from Chris, Karene and David to take your business and income to a totally different level, register on the link below and explore how you might be able to achieve your dreams much quicker than you thought by working together.

As successful business owners, we've coached and trained thousands of clients to success.

We're fortunate to make our living doing what we love, which is helping other experts to become successful.

But, it wasn't always easy. We all started out like most authors with no platform, no database, no experience, and a whole lot of questions. We spent many years figuring out how to sell books from scratch, build businesses, learn what works, and what doesn't. But you don't have to learn the hard way like we did. We're here to share with you what works and what doesn't so you can write and sell your expertise via books and increase your reputation and your income.

Take the next step in your Author Career and work with us directly. Click on the link below for more details about your next steps:

www.hcbpublishing.com

Work with us and learn how to use books to grow your

income and your business!

Printed in Great Britain
by Amazon

51368596R00093